Musculoskeletal Matters in Primary Care

Gill Wakley

Ruth Chambers

and

Paul Dieppe

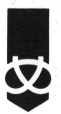

Staffordshire
UNIVERSITY

RADCLIFFE MEDICAL PRESS

Radcliffe Medical Press
18 Marcham Road, Abingdon, Oxon OX14 1AA

British Library Cataloguing in Publication Data

A catalogue record for this book is available from the British Library.

ISBN 1 85775 434 4

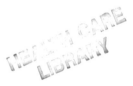

Typeset by Joshua Associates Ltd, Oxford
Printed and bound by TJ International Ltd, Padstow, Cornwall

Contents

About the authors

Gill Wakley started in general practice in 1966, but transferred to community medicine shortly afterwards and then into public health. A desire for increased contact with patients caused a move back into general practice, together with community gynaecology, in 1978. She has been combining the two, in varying amounts, ever since. She gained some experience of occupational health while working briefly for the Coal Board (including going underground), and personal encounters with arthritis have sharpened her awareness of the field.

Throughout she has been heavily involved in learning and teaching. She was in a training general practice, became an instructing doctor and a regional assessor in family planning, and was until recently a Senior Clinical Lecturer in the Primary Care Department at Keele University, Staffordshire. Like Ruth Chambers, she has run all types of educational initiatives and activities, from individual mentoring and instruction to small group work, plenary lectures, distance-learning programmes, workshops, and courses for a wide range of health professionals and lay people.

Ruth Chambers has been a GP for 20 years and is currently the Professor of Primary Care Development at Staffordshire University. She has undertaken a wide range of research and development focusing on stress and the health of doctors, health at work and the quality of healthcare. She has designed and organised many types of educational initiatives, including distance-learning programmes in occupational healthcare. Recently she has developed a keen interest in working with GPs, nurses and others in primary care around clinical governance and practice personal and professional development plans.

Paul Dieppe qualified in 1970, and has been a consultant rheumatologist since 1978. He was the Arthritis and Rheumatism Council Professor of Rheumatology at the University of Bristol between 1987 and 1997, when his particular research interest was osteoarthritis. He has been active in both public and professional educational initiatives in rheumatology.

Over the last few years his interests have broadened and he has become more concerned with disability issues and health services research. He is currently Director of the Medical Research Council's Health Services Research Collaboration, and is based in its lead centre in the Department of Social Medicine at the University of Bristol.

Glossary of common abbreviations and terms used

Case-control study	Each person in the study is matched (usually by at least age and sex) to one or more other individuals not exposed to the substance, illness or intervention being researched
Cohort study	A group of people being studied is matched to a group not exposed to that risk or suffering from that condition being studied
Critical incident analysis	The systematic analysis of a particular incident to establish beneficial or adverse effects on the outcome[1]
DEXA	Dual-energy X-ray absorptiometry
DMARD	Disease modifying anti-rheumatic drug
ESR	Erythrocyte sedimentation rate
GP	General practitioner
Guidelines	A written account of how a condition or intervention might be managed in the best way, customary way or to minimum standards.
Incidence	The frequency of first or new episodes of a condition in a defined population
Lupus	Contracted form of systemic lupus erythematosus
MRI	Magnetic resonance imaging
Meta-analysis	A statistical procedure to combine the results of several studies. However, it cannot correct for variations in quality or method of the original studies
NSAID	Non-steroidal anti-inflammatory drug
NSF	National Service Framework: the standards published by the Department of Health for the management of certain priority conditions
OA	osteoarthritis

Observational studies	Studies that look for associations between disease and exposure to known or suspected risk factors, or between interventions and progress of the disease
PDP	Personal development plan
PPDP	Practice, personal and professional development plan
Primary care organisation	Includes primary care trust, primary care group and local health groups
Placebo	An inactive intervention or substance used in a trial
Prevalence	The rate in a defined population of all cases of a condition, whether new or continuing
Protocol	A written set of rules for the management of a condition or for an intervention
RA	Rheumatoid arthritis
RCT	Randomised controlled trial, using two comparison groups selected by chance alone, one of which receives the intervention, while the other receives no intervention, a comparison intervention or placebo
Relative risk	One risk is given the score of unity (1) and other risks compared with it, or the ratio between the disease rate in people exposed to a risk factor and the rate in those not exposed to it
Shared care	When the management of a patient's condition is shared between health professionals from different disciplines or organisations
Significant event auditing	*See* critical incident analysis
Single group pre-post testing	A single group that has indicators required for the study recorded before and after exposure to the substance or intervention
SLE	Systemic lupus erythematosus
Systematic review	An academic research approach to reviewing the literature on a particular subject using guidelines to collect and grade all of the evidence on the subject[2]
Time series	Using a small group of people and following them up carefully over (usually) long periods of time to determine the outcome and modifying factors

Introduction

The material in this book sets out how learning more about musculo-skeletal disorders and reviewing current practice can be incorporated into the personal development plans of GPs, therapists, pharmacists, nurses or practice managers. There is a dual focus on best practice in the clinical management of musculoskeletal disorders and improving the working environment so that the practice systems and procedures are well organised. Practice team members should work together to direct their individual learning plans to form their practice personal and professional development plan, which complements the business plan of the practice, workplace or primary care organisation.

This programme is focused on musculoskeletal disorders because about one in seven patient visits to primary care are prompted by a musculoskeletal disorder.[3]

You may decide to allocate 50% of the time that you intend to spend drawing up, justifying and applying a personal development plan in any one year to best practice in musculoskeletal matters. That would leave space in your learning plan for other important topics such as mental health, coronary heart disease or cancer – whatever is a priority for you, your post and your patient population.

The first chapter of the book describes how a clinical governance culture incorporates good clinical management as well as environmental working conditions that are healthy and safe. You should be able to demonstrate that you are fit to practise as an individual clinician or manager (best practice in the management of musculoskeletal disorders), and that your working environment is fit to practise from (a well-organised practice). This section will be relevant to you whether you are a clinician, an employee or a manager, so that you understand more of the context within which you work and how your individual contribution fits into the whole picture of healthcare.

The chapters that follow provide important facts about the management of some of the more common or more serious musculoskeletal conditions, together with references so that you can find out more about particular subjects. Many changes in clinical management have occurred in recent years – for example, in the earlier use of disease-modifying drugs in rheumatoid arthritis, or in awareness of risk factors for osteoporosis. Back pain is not covered in this book, as it has a volume all to itself – *Back Pain Matters in Primary Care*.[4]

The material in the chapters that follow is designed to help to point you in the right direction in your search for information about musculoskeletal disorders. The whole programme builds up to enable you to create a personal development plan or practice personal and professional development plan in Chapters 13 and 14. Interactive exercises at the end of each chapter give you an opportunity to undertake an assessment of your learning needs, review your own performance or the efficiency of your practice organisation, and reflect on what improvements you could make.

You should transfer information from these needs assessment exercises to the relevant slots in the personal development plan if you are undertaking this programme as an individual, or to the practice personal and professional development plan if you are working as a team. Adopt a wide-based approach to improving quality – think of how you are establishing a clinical governance culture in your own practice team in your timed action plans.

What should you do next?

Study the template for a personal development plan on pages 123–132 or a practice personal and professional development plan on pages 123–153. You will be filling this in as you go along. Decide whether you will be starting out on your personal development plan or working with colleagues on the practice learning plan. You will need to ensure that each person's personal development plan meshes with the practice learning plan by the end.

Make changes as a result – to your workplace, or to the equipment in your practice, or to the advice that you give to patients, or to the way in which you manage and investigate musculoskeletal disorders or organise their prevention. Build in ways in which you can evaluate how well the changes have worked.

CHAPTER 1

Clinical governance and the management of musculoskeletal disorders

The range of musculoskeletal disorders is very wide, and overlaps occur between the specialties of rheumatology and orthopaedics, as well as between the many disciplines involved in caring for patients with these conditions. A selection of topics has been made to represent what might be of concern to a primary care team that is aiming to improve the management of this particular part of their workload.

Clinical governance is inclusive – making quality everyone's business, whether they are a doctor or a nurse, a pharmacist or other independent contractor, a manager, member of staff or a strategic planner. We need to know where we are now, and where we want to get to, if we are to drive up standards of healthcare.

Clinical governance involves doing 'anything and everything required to maximise quality'.[5,6] It should create a culture and working environment in which people thrive and feel fulfilled by their work but where, at the same time, under-performance is identified and corrected.

Components of clinical governance

The components of clinical governance are not new. However, bringing them together under the banner of clinical governance and introducing more explicit accountability for performance is a new style of working.

The following 14 themes are core components of professional and service development which, taken together, form a comprehensive approach to providing high-quality healthcare services and clinical governance.[5] These are illustrated in the tree diagram shown in Figure 1.1.

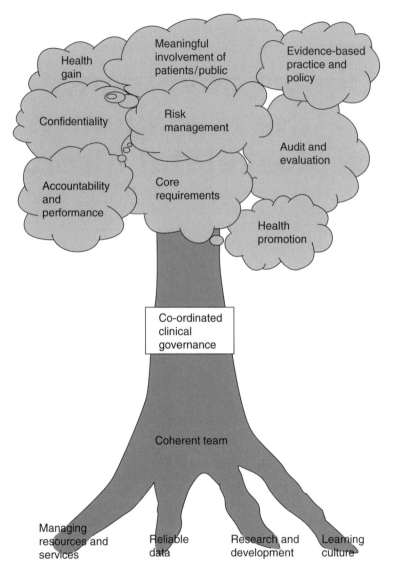

Figure 1.1: 'Routes' and branches of clinical governance.

If you interweave these components into your individual and workplace-based personal and professional development plans you will have addressed the requirements for clinical governance at the same time.[7]

1 *Learning culture*: in the practice, primary care organisation or department.
2 *Research and development culture*: in the practice or throughout the health service.

3 *Reliable and accurate data*: in the practice, and in the NHS as a seamless whole.

4 *Well-managed resources and services*: as individuals, as a practice, across the NHS and in conjunction with other organisations.

5 *Coherent team*: well-integrated teams within a practice, including attached staff.

6 *Meaningful involvement of patients and the public*: including users, carers and the general population.

7 *Health gain*: activities to improve the health of staff and patients within a practice, between practices, and in a primary care organisation.

8 *Confidentiality*: of information in consultations, in medical notes and between practitioners.

9 *Evidence-based practice and policy*: applying it in practice, in the district and across the NHS.

10 *Accountability and performance*: for standards, performance of individuals and the practice – both to the public and to those in authority.

11 *Core requirements*: good fit with skill mix and whether individuals are competent to do their jobs; communication, work-force numbers and morale at practice level.

12 *Health promotion*: for patients, the public, your staff and colleagues – both opportunistic and in general, targeting those with most needs.

13 *Audit and evaluation*: for instance, of the extent to which individuals and practice teams adhere to best practice in clinical management or human resources.

14 *Risk management*: being competent to spot those at risk; reducing risks and probabilities of ill health.

The challenges to delivering clinical governance

Delivering high-quality healthcare, with guaranteed minimum standards of care for users at all times, is a major challenge. At present the quality of healthcare is patchy and variable. We are not very good at detecting under-performance and then taking the initiative and rectifying it at an early stage. The small number of clinicians who do under-perform exert a disproportionately large effect on the public's confidence. Causes of under-performance in an individual might be a result of a lack of knowledge or skills, poor attitudes or ill health. The Arthritis Research Campaign have discussed the difficulties that some patients have experienced when consulting their doctors about arthritis. A news article on their website in October 2000 (*see* list of websites in the Appendix) gives two typical stories of lack of expertise shown by the doctors, and blames this on the lack of education at medical school. Although most medical schools now include rheumatology, it is reported that in five medical schools doctors had received no clinical rheumatology teaching at all. Most doctors who qualified a few years ago will not have had any rheumatology teaching, and will be in even more need of postgraduate learning. However, a lack of management capability is nearly always an important contributory factor to inadequate clinical services, and provision can be patchy.

We need to understand why variation exists and explore ways of reducing the inequalities. Variation in the quality of healthcare provided is common – between different practices in the same locality, between staff of the same discipline working in the same practice or unit, and between care given to some groups of the population rather than others. For example:

- the rates of referral to hospital may differ by fourfold between one doctor and another for the same condition
- some general practices have direct access to physiotherapists, whilst others have to refer patients to a hospital specialist first.

Clinical governance offers a co-ordinated approach to overcoming these areas of risk through a blend of clinical and organisational improvements in the quality of healthcare practice.

Learning culture

Education and training programmes should be relevant to service needs, whether at organisational or individual levels. Continuing professional development (CPD) programmes need to meet both the learning needs of individual health professionals and the wider service development needs of the NHS. You should no longer opt for CPD activities according to what you *want* to do, but rather according to what you *need* to do. Clinical governance underpins professional and service development.

> **Individual personal development plans**
> will feed into a
> **workplace or practice-based personal and**
> **professional development plan**
> that will feed into
> **the organisation's business plan**
> all of which are
> **underpinned by clinical governance.**[5]

Thus focusing on musculoskeletal disorders would be a good topic for a practice personal and professional development plan with a mix of learning about the effective clinical management of musculoskeletal disorders in a healthy and safe work environment.

Applying research and development in practice

The conclusions of the many thousands of research papers about musculoskeletal matters that are published in reputable journals each year are rarely applied in practice. This is because few health professionals or managers make time to read such journals systematically, and they are unaware of the research findings. Moreover, most practice teams do not have a system for reviewing important research papers and translating that review into practical action. The primary care organisation might help by feeding important new evidence to its constituent practices or pharmacies, the therapy units and clinics, or indeed the general public, with suggestions or templates for making changes in practice, backed by resources to enable change to occur.

Incorporating research-based evidence into everyday practice should promote policies on effective working, improve quality and expand the clinical governance culture.

> Research published in the 1980s challenged the accepted view at that time about the treatment of rheumatoid arthritis. This was that drugs were started for systematic relief, and then disease-modifying anti-rheumatic drugs (DMARDs) were added one by one, starting with the least toxic one. The new approach using

DMARDs early in the disease has proved very successful, but many primary care teams are unaware of this research and still delay the introduction of DMARDs if systematic relief is achieved by other means.

Reliable and accurate data

Clinicians, patients and administrators need reliable and accurate data to connect individuals or their healthcare records to other knowledge that is relevant to the care of the patient. Set the following standards for workplaces.

- Keep records in chronological order.
- Summarise medical records, within specified time period for records of new patients.
- Review dates for checks on medication, with audit in place to monitor adherence to standards and plan what to do about under-performance if necessary.
- Use computers for diagnostic recording.
- Record information from external sources (hospital, other organisations) that is relevant to individual patients or the workplace.

Keep good written records of policies and audits that relate to musculoskeletal disorders in the practice. An inspection at any time should show what audits have been undertaken and when, the changes in practice organisation that followed, the extent of staff training undertaken, and the future programme of monitoring.

Well-managed resources and services

The things you need to achieve best practice should be in the right place at the right time, and working correctly every time.
  Set standards in your workplace for:

- access to premises and availability of services for people with special needs, such as those with disability due to musculoskeletal disorders
- provision of routine and urgent appointments
- access to and provision for referral for investigation or treatment
- pro-active monitoring of chronic illness and disability
- alternatives to face-to-face consultations
- consultation length.

The six primary care services to which the public requires access are information, advice, triage and treatment, continuity of care, personal care and other services.[8]

Systems should be designed to prevent and detect errors. Therefore keep systems simple and sensible, and inform everyone how those systems operate, so that they are less likely to bypass the system or make errors. This certainly applies to follow-up of patients' clinical management.

Coherent teamwork

Teams produce better patient care than single practitioners operating in a fragmented way. Effective teams make the most of the different contributions of individual clinical disciplines in delivering patient care. The characteristics of effective teams include the following:

- shared ownership of a common purpose
- clear goals for the contributions that each discipline makes
- open communication between team members
- opportunities for team members to enhance their skills.

A team approach helps different team members to adopt an evidence-based approach to patient care – by having to justify their approach to the rest of the team.[9]

Musculoskeletal disorders are conditions that require teamwork to achieve the best results for individual patients. The primary care team may include GPs and practice nurses, physiotherapists, occupational therapists, non-clinical staff and community pharmacists, and often extends to include shared care with secondary care services.

Meaningful involvement of patients and the public

People use terms such as 'user' or 'consumer' to describe who we should be involving in giving us feedback about the quality or type of healthcare that we offer, or in planning future services. Patients or carers, non-users of services, the local community, a particular subgroup of the population or the general public will all have useful feedback and views – for example, on the safety of your own practice premises, or your systems that inform patients' about the results of investigations or queries.

If user involvement and public participation are done well they should result in the following:

- reductions in health inequalities
- better outcomes of individual care
- better health of the population
- better quality and more locally responsive services
- greater ownership of health services
- a better understanding of why and how local services need to be changed and developed.

A meaningful public consultation involves the exchange of information between the healthcare providers and the general public. As a result, a representative opinion is obtained that feeds into the local decision-making process of healthcare services or whoever is sponsoring the consultation.

You might want to consult the public and health professionals about the availability of complementary therapies or exercise 'on prescription'. Alternatively, you could select a group of representative patients to help to educate healthcare staff about the problems faced by those affected by musculoskeletal disorders.

Representative opinions may be difficult or expensive to obtain. You may have to trade off a relatively cheaper method of consultation that engages with fewer people or with a less representative section of the population subgroup. If you do, you will need to understand what biases are arising and make allowances for those biases when you interpret the results of the consultation.[10]

Health gain

The two general approaches to improving health are the 'population' approach, which focuses on measures to improve health through the community, and the 'high-risk' approach, which focuses on vulnerable individuals who are at high risk of the condition or hazard.

The two approaches are not mutually exclusive, and they often need to be combined with legislation and community action. Health goals include the following:

- a good quality of life
- avoiding premature death
- equal opportunities for health.

Modifiable risk factors for reducing the adverse effects of musculo-skeletal disorders include the following:

- obesity
- lack of exercise
- occupational or sporting hazards.

Confidentiality

Confidentiality is a component of clinical governance that is often overlooked. Experienced health professionals and managers may assume that junior or new staff know all about confidentiality, and of course they may not. There are many difficult situations in the work-place where one person asks for information about another's medical condition (e.g. test results or a progress report) and it is not clear-cut whether this information should be supplied or withheld. Sometimes it is not even clear whether the person who is asked should acknowledge that the person being enquired about is under their care.

The Caldicott Committee Report describes the following principles of good practice to safeguard confidentiality when information is being used for non-clinical purposes.[11]

- Justify the purpose.
- Do not use patient-identifiable information unless it is absolutely necessary to do so.
- Use the minimum necessary patient-identifiable information.
- Access to patient-identifiable information should be on a strict need-to-know basis.
- Everyone with access to patient-identifiable information should be aware of his or her responsibilities.

Evidence-based culture

Protocols have come to have a specific meaning in the health service. The purpose of a protocol is to direct healthcare staff along preferred pathways by outlining detailed management plans for discrete (usually clinical) conditions. These conditions are judged to be suitable for step-wise decision-making processes that can be specified in flow diagrams or algorithms.[12] Protocols are considered to be more restrictive than guidelines, and their relevance to clinical situations is limited to certain specific occasions when their rigidity of purpose minimises risk. They are often used when treatment is delegated to staff who would not otherwise have this responsibility and who do not have the knowledge or training to deviate from the protocol.

Guidelines are a collection of recommendations that embody certain standards of management. These standards are (or should be) based on evidence and may:

- set out minimum reasonable standards
- codify customary standards
- recommend best practice.

Recommendations are usually less strongly worded than guidelines, and may be based on less certain evidence. Sometimes they are used almost interchangeably with guidelines, but they often imply recommended action suggested by an expert (or committee of experts) to non-experts.

Codes of practice usually imply not only guidelines on safety and efficacy, but also ethical and social aspects of the problem.

Practice policies consist of agreed courses of action (or guidelines), in particular clinical or non-clinical situations. They direct the healthcare staff to take certain actions for groups of patients or for individuals. They tend to be reached by consensus after discussion of various options, considering the consequences of those options and deciding on the desirability of particular outcomes for patients.[13]

The evidence for protocols and guidelines

There are several systems of grading evidence. A classification[14] that is often quoted gives the strength of evidence as follows.

Strength of evidence

Type I: Strong evidence from at least one systematic review of multiple well-designed randomised controlled trials (RCTs).

Type II: Strong evidence from at least one properly designed RCT of appropriate size.

Type III: Evidence from well-designed trials without randomisation, single-group pre–post, cohort, time-series or matched case–control studies.

Type IV: Evidence from well-designed non-experimental studies from more than one centre or research group.

Type V: The opinions of respected authorities, based on clinical evidence, descriptive studies or reports of expert committees.

Other categories of evidence[15] are listed in the compendium of the best available evidence for effective healthcare, *Clinical Evidence*, which is updated every six months, and is perhaps more useful to the health professional in everyday work.

Beneficial:	Interventions whose effectiveness has been shown by clear evidence from controlled trials.
Likely to be beneficial:	Interventions for which effectiveness is less well established than for those listed under 'beneficial'.
Trade-off between benefits and harm:	Interventions for which clinicians and patients should weigh up the beneficial and harmful effects according to individual circumstances and priorities.
Unknown effectiveness:	Interventions for which there are currently insufficient data or data of inadequate quality (including interventions that are widely accepted as beneficial but which have never been formally tested in RCTs, often because the latter would be regarded as unethical).
Unlikely to be beneficial:	Interventions for which lack of effectiveness is less well established than for those listed under 'likely to be ineffective or harmful'.
Likely to be ineffective or harmful:	Interventions whose ineffectiveness or harmfulness has been demonstrated by clear evidence.

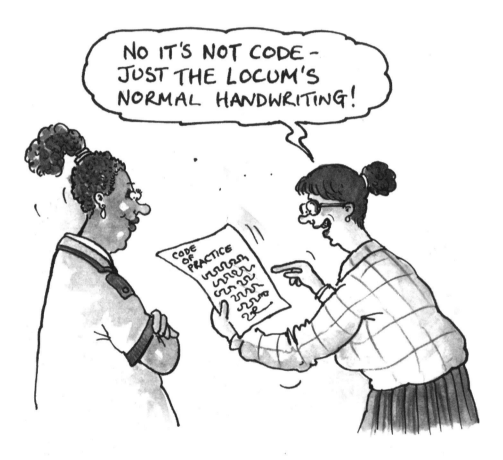

Using guidelines

The key features that determined whether or not local guidelines worked in one initiative[16] were as follows.

- There was multidisciplinary involvement in drawing them up.
- A well-described systematic review of the literature underpinned the guidelines, with graded recommendations for best practice linked to the evidence.
- Ownership was nurtured at both national and local levels.
- A local implementation plan ensured that all of the practicalities (time, staff, education and training, and resources) were foreseen and met, stakeholders were supported, and predictors of sustainability were addressed (guideline usability, and individualising guidelines to practitioners and patients).

Guidelines on the prevention and treatment of osteoporosis were drawn up in 1999 by the Royal College of Physicians,[17] and were updated by the Bone and Tooth Society in 2000.[18] The guidance lists the grades of evidence for the effectiveness of the options for the prevention and treatment of bone loss and fracture at various sites.

Accountability and performance

Health professionals may not always realise that they are accountable to others from outside their own professions, especially those with self-employed status such as GPs and pharmacists. In fact they are accountable to the following:

- the general public, who are entitled to expect high standards of healthcare
- the profession – to maintain standards of knowledge and skills of the profession as a whole
- the government – and employer – who expect high standards of healthcare from the workforce.

Health professionals who believe that they are not accountable to others may be reluctant to collect the evidence to demonstrate that they are fit to practise, and that their working environment is fit to practise from. They may be reluctant to co-operate with central NHS requirements, such as working to the National Service Frameworks.

Identify and rectify under-performance at an early stage by:

- regular appraisals (at least annually) linked to clinical governance and personal development plans. Appraisal is a process of regular meetings between manager and staff member, or doctor or pharmacist, with an external appraiser, with support for the benefit of the person who is being appraised
- detecting those who have significant health problems and referring them for help
- systematic audit that detects individuals' performance, as opposed to the overall performance of the practice team
- an open learning culture in which team members are discouraged from covering up colleagues' inadequacies, so that problems can be resolved at an early stage.

Clinicians may regard the performance assessment framework as a management tool that is not particularly relevant to their clinical practice. However, it does reinforce a clinical governance culture whereby good clinical management and organisational management have a symbiotic relationship.

The NHS performance assessment framework has six components, namely health improvement, fair access, efficiency, effective delivery of appropriate care, user/carer experience and health outcomes.

Health promotion

People may underestimate relative risks as applied to themselves and their own behaviour. For example, many smokers accept the relationship between smoking tobacco and disease, but do not believe that they personally are at risk. People usually have a reasonable idea of the *relative* risks of various activities and behaviours, although their personal estimates of the *magnitude* of those risks tend to be biased – small probabilities are often over-estimated and high probabilities are often under-estimated.

> Many people accept that they are overweight and inactive but do not make the link between that and the pain in their knees. Published research[19] has suggested that exercise alone, and exercise combined with weight loss, can both reduce pain and disability and improve performance in older obese people with knee osteoarthritis.

Audit and evaluation

Audit will probably be the method you think of first for determining your needs – as a clinician or as a practice. You might look at the extent to which you are adhering to practice or pharmacy protocols – for instance, whether you are consistently advising those with musculo-skeletal disorders to remain active, or comparing other aspects of clinical care with best-practice guidelines. You might monitor delay between the provisional diagnosis of rheumatoid arthritis and the time of prescription of disease-modifying drugs, or the number of musculoskeletal injuries that occur among staff over a 12-month period.

> The shared care between hospital and general practice using protocols to monitor the use of disease-modifying drugs in rheu-matoid arthritis was audited.[20] This audit showed that the ideal protocol was followed in 93% of cases for methotrexate, but in only 26% of cases for gold. The main difficulties were associated with specimen transfer or due to communication failures between hospital, patient and the general practice.

Analysis of critical or significant incidents should focus on organisational factors, not just on the performance of particular individuals.

A patient taking non-steroidal anti-inflammatory drugs for osteoarthritis has a haematemesis. Review of the notes shows that she had a history of reflux oesophagitis two years previously, but that this had not been recorded in her record summary. She had never attended for the endoscopy, and had said that she was better, so it was not recorded as a definite diagnosis. In order to reduce the likelihood of this occurring again, reminder prompts to ask 'Any history of indigestion?' were added to the screen that appeared when non-steroidal anti-inflammatory drugs were to be prescribed.

Core requirements

You cannot deliver clinical governance without well-trained and competent staff, the right skill mix of staff, a safe and comfortable working environment, and the provision of cost-effective care. Following published referral guidelines may increase healthcare costs, and these should be justifiable as cost-effective care when all direct and indirect costs are taken into account.

Your healthcare team can do much under the umbrella of clinical governance to respond to the government challenges to improve the following:

- *partnership*: working together across the NHS to ensure the best possible care
- *performance*: acting to review and deliver higher standards of healthcare
- *the professions and wider work-force*: breaking down barriers between different disciplines (e.g. through multidisciplinary teamwork between GPs and nurses with pharmacists)
- *patient care*: access, convenient services, and empowerment to take a full part in decision making about their own medical care and in planning and providing health services in general
- *prevention*: promoting healthy living across all sections of society, and tackling variations in care.

Risk management

Risk management in general practice mainly centres on assessing probabilities that potential or actual hazards will give rise to harm – how bad the risk is, how likely it is that the risk will occur, when the risk will occur (if ever) and how certain are you of estimates about the risks. This applies just as much whether the risk is an environmental or organisational risk within the practice, or a clinical risk.

> A member of staff is off sick with wrist tendinitis following long periods of work at a keyboard, and another staff member is off sick with a sprained ankle after stepping off a kick stool used to reach notes above head height. A risk assessment and analysis of the workplace reveals several areas where changes might reduce potential hazards and prevent a recurrence. Look at *Occupational Health Matters in General Practice* for other examples.[21]

Good practice means understanding and managing risk – both clinical and organisational aspects. Undertaking audit more systematically will reduce the risks of omission both in detection and in clinical management. The common areas of risk in providing healthcare services are thought to include the following:[22]

- out-of-date clinical practice
- lack of continuity of care
- poor communication
- mistakes in patient care
- patient complaints
- financial risk – insufficient resources
- reputation
- staff morale.

Communicating and managing risks with individual patients is very much about finding ways to explain risks and elicit people's values and preferences so that all of these dimensions can be incorporated into the decisions that they themselves make – to take risks or choose between alternatives that involve different risks and benefits. A well-functioning system through which patients can make complaints and receive feedback on the outcome should allow the practice or unit to reduce risks of a recurrence.

An obese patient with diabetes developed a frozen shoulder. After poor progress with physiotherapy, the GP agreed to inject the shoulder with a corticosteroid. Unfortunately, the patient developed an infected joint, septicaemia, and died. Her family made an informal complaint directly to the doctor, but were surprisingly understanding when a full explanation of the relative risks was given and they were shown a record of the discussion of the risks in the patient's record. The doctor was very glad that he had learned from a previous complaint how to present the balance of risks in a way that was comprehensible.

Make sure that the clinicians who are responsible for joint injection in your practice or primary care organisation (PCO) are competent and up to date.

Reflection exercise

Exercise 1

Review and plan to improve your knowledge, attitudes and skills with regard to musculoskeletal disorders

Any member or members of the practice team might consider how to integrate the 14 components of clinical governance into their personal development plan. Examples are given for each component listed below. Try to complete this from your own perspective.

- *Establishing a learning culture:* e.g. arrange a session to update staff at a multidisciplinary meeting on guidelines and up-to-date information about the management of musculoskeletal disorders.
- *Managing resources and services:* e.g. inform primary care organisations about shortfalls in physiotherapy services, or the poor availability of secondary care facilities; arrange for nurse-run shared care protocols for chronic disease management.
- *Establishing a research and development culture:* e.g. undertake some original research into musculoskeletal disorders, perhaps by linking with your local university; share published papers citing evidence on musculoskeletal disorders with work colleagues.

- *Reliable and accurate data:* e.g. record musculoskeletal disorders in a clear and consistent way so that you can repeat the exercise next year and compare the results.
- *Evidence-based practice and policy:* e.g. formulate a protocol for prescribing or referring for musculoskeletal disorders.
- *Confidentiality:* e.g. take care with whom you share information from medical records; develop policies for giving results of investigations.
- *Health gain:* e.g. target patients with other medical conditions who are most vulnerable to the adverse effects of osteoporosis or osteoarthritis.
- *Coherent team:* e.g. communicate new systems and procedures effectively between all members of your team.
- *Audit and evaluation:* e.g. undertake regular audits and act on the findings to improve quality.
- *Meaningful involvement of patients and the public:* e.g. listen to and act on patients' comments about your clinical care or your services; use patient support groups.
- *Health promotion:* e.g. promote weight control and accident prevention among practice staff; obtain or write leaflets about the prevention of musculoskeletal disorders.
- *Accountability and performance:* e.g. keep good records to demonstrate your own good practice.
- *Core requirements:* e.g. agree on roles and responsibilities in the team for the various practice policies and tasks.
- *Risk management:* e.g. establish systems and procedures to identify, analyse and minimise the risks, such as during repeat prescribing, over-investigation, unsafe working practices.

Now that you have completed the interactive reflection exercise in this chapter, transfer the information from this needs assessment to the empty templates. Use the personal development plan on pages 123–132 if you are working on your own learning plan, or the practice personal and professional development plan on pages 147–153 if you are working on a practice team learning plan. The conclusions reached at the end of each exercise will feature in the action plan. Don't forget to keep the evidence of your learning in your personal portfolio.

CHAPTER 2

Managing the initial presentation of musculoskeletal disorders

You can sort out most disorders that present for the first time in primary care with a competent history and physical examination. Avoid diagnostic tests unless they will aid your management or you need them for a baseline. Be prepared to assess the patient again later when the diagnosis may be clearer.

The history

Your most important task is to ensure that you identify serious conditions which need urgent evaluation. There are three types of condition that you do not want to miss – malignancy, bone or joint sepsis, and major vessel or nerve damage – so look out for the 'red flags' which suggest that one or other of these conditions may be present (*see* Table 2.1). In addition, check for a history of serious trauma, which can result in fractures or unstable joints.[3]

Assessing pain

Pain is the main presenting symptom of musculoskeletal disorders. In general, the history will give you a good idea of the type of musculo-skeletal pathology that is present, and in particular whether the pain is inflammatory or mechanical in nature, whereas an examination is necessary to establish the anatomical source of the pain.[23]

It is helpful to know the character of the pain, where it is, and what makes it better or worse.

Table 2.1 'Red flags' that require urgent action

Condition	Symptoms and signs
Sepsis	Hot swollen joint, fever, redness over a very tender bone or joint, general malaise, weight loss
Malignancy	General ill health, malaise, weight loss, severe constant pain in bones, that is not affected by rest or exercise
Neurovascular damage	Burning pain radiating in a nerve or nerve-root distribution, claudication, cold white extremities, sensory or motor loss

- Pain that is described as numbness, burning, shooting or 'pins and needles' may be neurological, especially if its distribution is localised to a dermatome, peripheral nerve or a stocking-glove type.
- Claudication pain from arterial insufficiency occurs during use and is relieved by rest. Lumbar spinal stenosis neurogenic pain presents with pain on walking that is relieved slowly by sitting or spinal flexion.
- Pain from articular structures is usually worse on movement or weight bearing, and is relieved by rest.
- Pain that is vaguely localised to a joint, but where the joint appears normal, may be due to referred pain or a bone lesion. Bone lesions often cause unceasing night pain.
- Prolonged morning stiffness in multiple painful joints and some improvement with exercise usually indicates an inflammatory rheumatic condition such as rheumatoid arthritis (RA). These symptoms may be accompanied by feeling ill, fever, weight loss, and signs and symptoms of involvement of other parts of the body, such as dry eyes and mouth, rashes, red eyes, urethritis, adenopathy, oral ulcers, pleuritic chest pain or Raynaud's phenomenon.
- Morning stiffness of shorter duration with little or no pain at rest, and with pain increasing during or after sustained exercise, suggests local mechanical problems (bursitis, tendinitis, sprains or strains) or osteoarthritis (OA), especially if there is no systemic illness.

Regional musculoskeletal pain has three main causes:

- periarticular lesions, such as tendinitis, bursitis and enthesopathies (problems at ligament or tendon insertions)
- mechanical problems with joints, such as internal derangements or osteoarthritis
- inflammatory synovitis.

Table 2.2 Useful clinical features when evaluating a patient with musculoskeletal pain

	Periarticular problem	OA or internal derangement	Inflammatory rheumatic disease
Symptoms			
Morning stiffness	Usually absent	Local, short-lived	Severe and prolonged
Time when it is worse	With use	With use	After prolonged inactivity
General ill health	Not relevant	Not relevant	Often present
Locking or instability	Uncommon (only with tendinitis)	Implies a loose body, internal derangement or weakness	Uncommon in early disease, may result from late joint damage
Symmetry	Uncommon	Occasional	Usual
Signs			
Tenderness	Focal, periarticular (or tender points in fibromyalgia)	Over a single joint line	Over the joint line of all affected joints
Inflammation (fluid, warmth)	Occasionally over tendon or bursa	Absent or mild	Severe
Other systems involved	No	No	Sometimes

Clues that are helpful when assessing pain are shown in Table 2.2.

It is important to find out what disability may result from the condition. Lower limb problems may cause walking difficulties, and upper limb problems may cause difficulty with reaching and dexterity. So, useful questions to ask include the following.

1 'Do you have any difficulty climbing stairs?' (if a patient can climb stairs and steps, he or she can walk and get on buses).
2 'Do you have any difficulty washing or dressing yourself?' (impairments of dexterity, reaching and personal care are common, and washing and dressing are among the most important tasks to be affected).

In addition, other impairments may make things much worse, so it is always worth asking about sensory problems such as problems with sight or hearing, especially in older people.

Psychosocial factors are important. Pain and the loss of ability to do tasks that could previously be achieved are depressing, and cause anxiety and loss of self-esteem. This in turn makes the pain more difficult to bear. Occupation may be an important factor, as many common musculoskeletal problems are over-use injuries.

Physical examination

Look for the signs listed in Table 2.2 above. The following may also help with diagnosis.

1 *Warmth over the joint*: this suggests an inflammatory process (beware of the recently removed bandage or hot-water bottle).
2 *Joint swelling*: this may be due to an effusion in the joint, synovial thickening, bony enlargement (as with osteophytes) or oedema in the surrounding tissues. Effusion suggests synovitis.
3 *Pain on movement of the joint*:
   - point tenderness, reduced active range of movement and preserved passive range of movement – may be due to soft tissue periarticular disorder, including bursitis, tendinitis and muscle injury
   - both active and passive movements limited – may be due to soft tissue contracture, synovitis or a structurally abnormal joint
   - tenderness along the course of a tendon, or pain or a rub produced when put on the stretch – may be due to tendinitis
   - unable to abduct the shoulder fully – may be due to rotator cuff damage
   - crepitus with pain (ignore if without pain) – may be due to articular surface abnormalities.
4 *An unstable knee or ankle without muscle weakness*: this suggests a ligament tear.
5 Look for general signs that are suggestive of conditions such as the scaly patches of psoriasis, or the butterfly facial rash of systemic lupus erythematosus.
6 Look for general systemic signs if the history suggests a systemic rheumatoid illness or a connective tissue disorder.

Arthralgia, with or without myalgia, without any physical signs can be very difficult to diagnose when you see it first. Plan to reassess rather than launching into diagnostic testing, which is usually unhelpful.

Causes of arthralgia include the following:

- fibromyalgia
- neuropathy
- viral infection
- hypothyroidism
- overuse syndrome
- metabolic bone disease (rare).

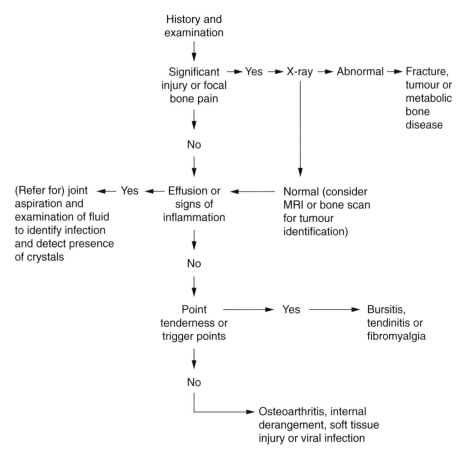

Figure 2.1: Flow chart for recognising patterns of musculoskeletal disorders when one or a few joints are affected.

Myalgia alone is common. It can be secondary to a localised problem (e.g. injury or overuse), or to a more general systemic illness (e.g. infection, toxic or metabolic disorders). Occasionally it may be a primary muscle disease. Consider fibromyalgia in an otherwise healthy patient with normal strength and multiple tender points. Proximal

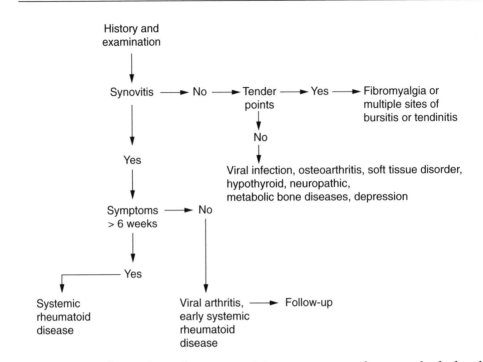

Figure 2.2: Flow chart for recognising patterns of musculoskeletal disorders when many joints are affected.

weakness (and a raised creatinine level) suggests an inflammatory myopathy.

Consider polymyalgia rheumatica in any patient over 50 years of age with myalgia of the hip or shoulder girdle, and check the erythrocyte sedimentation rate (ESR).

Investigations

If after the history and examination you conclude that the problem is a mechanical or extra-articular one, then investigations are unnecessary. Beware of performing investigations without considering what you will do with the results. Abnormalities are often found in the absence of disease, especially as people grow older.

If you are unsure what tests are currently indicated, ask your laboratory for help, or consult an up-to-date reference guide.[24]

An ESR is non-specific, but it is useful if you suspect an infection, inflammation or malignancy. A very high ESR suggests polymyalgia rheumatica, giant-cell arteritis or cancer.

Table 2.3

Diagnosis suspected	Investigation
Viral arthritis	Hepatitis serology; Lyme or parvovirus, or other viral studies
Myositis with muscle weakness	Creatinine phosphokinase; myositis-specific antibodies
Spondylitis	HLA-B27
Wegener's granulomatosis	Antineutrophil cytoplasmic antibody

Only request rheumatoid factor (RF) and/or antinuclear antibody (ANA) tests if you suspect a systemic rheumatoid disease. The higher the level of RF, the more likely it is that the diagnosis is rheumatoid arthritis (RA), but at least 25% of patients with RA never have a raised RF level. Other inflammatory conditions such as systemic lupus erythematosus (SLE) or viral infections may also show a positive RF. A high titre of ANA makes SLE more likely, but false-positive test results often occur.

In patients with multisystem symptoms and signs, full blood count and biochemical screening to include liver and kidney function is usually undertaken. Other, more sophisticated tests can be performed for specific diagnostic possibilities (*see* Table 2.3).

In *acute* gout, levels of uric acid may not be raised. The level is more useful for monitoring medication in order to control a raised level found between attacks with the typical symptoms and signs of gout.

Synovial fluid requires examination in an acutely inflamed single joint in order to rule out infection, and can be useful for distinguishing other types of effusion or synovitis. For example, you might need to use it to differentiate pseudogout (in which calcium or crystal deposits fall out of the cartilage into the joint and cause synovial inflammation) from other causes of a red swollen knee.

X-rays

Plain radiographs are not helpful for most patients who you think have acute or new symptoms and signs of RA, SLE, gout, mechanical back pain, tendinitis or bursitis. They may confirm the presence of osteoarthritis, but can be normal in the early stages.

Imaging is indicated if you have a history of significant injury, if joint function is lost, if pain continues despite conservative management, or if there is a history of malignancy. A bone scan is useful if osteomyelitis or malignancy are suspected. Magnetic resonance imaging (MRI) should be reserved for patients in whom a specific abnormality is suspected.

Management of acute musculoskeletal conditions

Most acute conditions are due to injury or over-use and do not require any investigations. You could look at the 'Ottowa rules' for sets of clinical decision rules about the use of X-rays in injuries. They list ankle and knee injuries so far (*see Bandolier* website in the Appendix for useful reviews of these articles), and would help you to set the standards if you wished to audit the use of X-rays in these conditions.

Acute injuries and sprains are usually treated according to the acronym **RICE**:

- *Rest*: only until the swelling and the worst of the pain have subsided.
- *Ice*: ice-packs (with the skin protected from ice-burns) or alternate cold and hot bathing reduce the swelling. Warn patients to test the temperature before immersing in hot or cold water or applying the hot or cold pad!
- *Compression*: 'support' might be a better term, but does not fit so well in the acronym. A sling or double tubigrip bandage will support a tennis elbow, and a firm figure-of-eight elastic bandage will support a sprained ankle. Strap one finger to another for an over-extension injury. Remember to allow for an increase in swelling in the immediate post-injury period, and do not use continuously for more than a few days or muscle weakness will complicate the recovery.
- *Elevation*: reduce the swelling by avoiding dependent positions for the affected part. A sprained ankle will be much more comfortable if it is placed well above the level of the pelvis.

Some patients will want to use pain relief (e.g. ibuprofen or paracetamol), but others prefer to be aware of the recovery rate and when mobilisation can be started.

Start gradual mobilisation as soon as possible. Gradual non-weight-bearing stretching exercises are usually advised after 4–5 days. Exercise in warm water is ideal if possible, as the water supports the injured part. Physiotherapists, especially those with an interest in sports physiotherapy, are a good resource for expert advice on how to return function to normal as quickly as possible. Leaflets on what to do will help some patients, and some useful ones on common conditions (e.g. tennis elbow) are available from the Arthritis and Rheumatism Council (*see* the Appendix for a list of useful addresses).

Referral

Ideally referral should take place after discussion and agreement between the patient and the doctor for specific purposes. A referral should be considered:

- when specialised investigations are needed, e.g. joint aspiration and examination
- when specialised medical treatment is needed, e.g. steroids or immunosuppressive drugs
- when specialised surgical treatment is needed, e.g. tendon or muscle tears, fractures, joint replacement
- when the condition is not controlled or diagnosed after management in primary care
- when the patient or their family are very anxious or ask for a specialist referral.

An Arthritis Research Campaign booklet[25] on referral guidelines for general practitioners gives a useful list of what a rheumatologist has to offer:

For diagnosis, they can offer:

- skill with musculoskeletal examination
- synovial fluid analysis
- interpretation of immunological tests
- access to special imaging modalities
- tissue biopsy techniques
- experience of rare rheumatic disorders.

For management, they can offer:

- skills in counselling arthritis patients
- education and self-help programmes
- a therapeutic team of professions allied to medicine (physiotherapy, occupational therapy, specialist nurses, etc.)
- admission for ill patients
- ability to aspirate or inject any joint
- specialist knowledge of immunosuppressive drug regimes
- ability to assess activity and progress

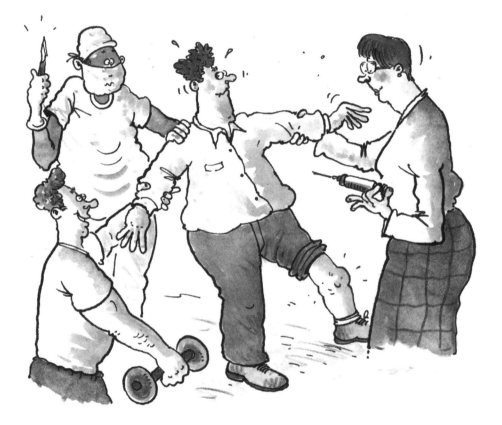

- access to combined orthopaedic clinics
- experience with rare complications
- special therapeutic interventions.

Shared care

If a shared care plan between specialists and general practice does not exist, consider setting one up. The ARC booklet[25] contains a useful outline. Remember to send all of *your* findings to the specialist when referring or after any significant change in management. Electronic records make this sharing much more flexible. Those with access to a suitable machine can read Smart Cards (like a credit card but containing personal medical details as digital information) with different levels of access depending on need. Patients, specialists and general practitioners can download centrally accessible records holding electronic information with suitable safeguards for identification of the user. Until these methods are more generally available, a patient-held card might contain the following information:

- patient identification
- relevant diagnosis
- key investigation results
- current management plan for self-care, physical therapy and exercises, daily living advice and medication
- changes that require action (what to do if the condition flares up, what to watch for with the medication, what to do if the disability worsens)
- contacts and enquiry telephone numbers, e.g. arthritis support nurse, hospital contact, etc.

Reflection exercises

Exercise 2

As a practice team/doctor/physiotherapist/practice nurse, you might review the practice protocol or guidelines for managing the diagnosis of musculoskeletal disorders

If your practice does not have these yet, now is the time to get together a small representative group to set them up. You might want to involve other colleagues (e.g. doctors, practice nurses, physiotherapists, osteopaths, chiropractors) in their development and use. You might want to adapt the flow charts in Figures 2.1 and 2.2, for example, or look for already established guidelines that you can modify for local use.

Exercise 3

As a doctor/physiotherapist/practice nurse, you might:

(i) Set up a clinical updating meeting to make sure that everyone clinically involved knows about the importance of 'red flags', or add a warning on the computer to be triggered automatically, or do both.
(ii) List some common clinical presentations and circulate them at coffee-time to see how many variations of 'labels' for the condition you can obtain. Then check against the diagnostic codes used in your workplace, and reach a consensus with your practice colleagues so that data is entered in a consistent way.

   This makes it much easier to check whether any interventions that are made alter the management of those conditions.

Exercise 4

As a practice manager/member of reception staff/secretary, you might check to see whether non-clinical staff are entering diagnoses from secondary care letters and discharge notes from a list of 'approved diagnostic codes'. This list needs to be the same as that used by the clinical staff, so reach a consensus if you are drawing up a new list. The codes you use in your practice are unlikely to be the same as those that are used throughout the primary care organisation, so think about how they could be harmonised to provide better baseline data. The practice manager may wish to make representations to the primary care organisation for help with this project.

Exercise 5

As a practice manager/audit receptionist/doctor/clinical governance lead, you might take a sample of patients referred for hip, knee and ankle X-rays (and/or shoulder, elbow and wrist X-rays). The sample could be a time sample, e.g. everyone for the next 8 weeks. You could use a random sample (consider having one stratified for age and sex) generated by the computer from a total search of all patients who have had a referral of this type in the last 12 months. (You might identify some other learning needs in the process for learning about randomisation or how to set up searches on the computer system.) Audit whether the recommendations for imaging (*see* above) have been followed. Decide how to take action if you find that many patients are being referred for X-rays inappropriately – you might want to present the findings at a practice team meeting, or circulate each referrer and ask for comments. Build in a time (perhaps 6 months) when you will repeat the audit after any necessary changes have been implemented, and remember to give feedback to those who have had to make the changes. If this action has worked well, consider passing on the details to your primary care organisation so that other practices (and patients) can benefit, too.

Now that you have completed one or more of the interactive reflection exercises in this chapter, transfer the information from this needs assessment to the empty templates. Use the personal development plan on pages 123–132 if you are working on your own learning plan, or the practice personal and professional development plan on pages 147–153 if you are working on a practice team learning plan. The conclusions reached at the end of each exercise will feature in the action plan. Don't forget to keep the evidence of your learning in your personal portfolio.

CHAPTER 3

Osteoarthritis

What is osteoarthritis?

Osteoarthritis is a heterogeneous condition that varies according to the joints affected with regard to its prevalence, risk factors, clinical features and prognosis. It most commonly affects the knees, hips, spinal apophyseal joints and the hands. It is usually defined by the pathological or radiological appearance of the joints, rather than by the clinical features. Characteristically the cartilage surfaces of synovial joints show focal areas of damage together with remodelling of the underlying bone and mild synovitis. In severely affected joints, the joint space is narrowed and osteophytes form, with visible radiological subchondral bone changes.

How common is osteoarthritis?

People usually start to develop osteoarthritis between the ages of 45 and 55 years, and the prevalence of the condition increases with age. Only 5% of people below the age of 40 years will have any evidence of osteoarthritis,[26] rising to 70% by the age of 75 years. It is three times as common in women as in men. The knee is the commonest site and affects 10% of the population over 50 years of age. Osteoarthritis of the hip is less common than that of the knee, at less than 3% up to the age of 65 years, increasing to 5% in people over 80 years of age.

Clinical features

Currently, diagnosis is made on the basis of the structural changes detected either clinically or by the X-ray appearance. There is often a discrepancy between the radiographic appearance and the symptoms. The challenge for health professionals is to determine the extent to which the radiographic changes (so commonly present in people over the age of 60 years) are contributing to the patient's overall problems. A possible scheme for the assessment of the current clinical picture is shown in Box 3.1. Look at the general assessment of musculoskeletal disease in Chapter 2 as well, and remember that just because someone has osteoarthritis, you cannot ignore the possibility of other coexisting musculoskeletal disorders.

Box 3.1 Assessment of patients: are the symptoms associated with the osteoarthritis or with other conditions in a patient who happens to have osteoarthritis?

(*see* Chapter 2 for differential diagnostic clues)

Type of pain
- Mechanical: does it improve or worsen after use? (in osteoarthritis, pain is worse with use)
- Inflammatory: for how long do stiffness and pain after rest last? (in osteoarthritis they are usually short-lived)
- Is night pain present? (If it is severe, consider metastases or infection)

Ask about other symptoms
- Sleep disturbance (if present, establish whether it is due to the pain, or consider depression or fibromyalgia)
- Joint locking (often present with a loose body, internal derangement or muscle weakness)
- Loss of function (consider nerve or muscle conditions)
- Is there a previous history of a precipitating cause, such as joint injury or disease (rather than osteoarthritis)?

Examination
- Is the pain in the joint or around it? (Consider peri-articular disease)
- Are there painful points in the muscles as well? (Consider fibromyalgia)

Management

The aims of treatment are as follows:

- patient education
- control of pain
- improvement of function and quality of life
- avoidance of adverse effects of treatment
- minimising progression.

The Primary Care Rheumatology Society has drawn up guidelines on the management of osteoarthritis (see list of useful addresses in the Appendix, and sources of guidelines[27]).

Non-drug therapies

Non-drug therapies for osteoarthritis are listed in Box 3.2, and referral to physiotherapists, orthotists and occupational therapists, as well as to social support agencies, can be extremely effective in improving function and lessening pain. For example, attending a day centre may enable a patient to eat more wisely, reduce depression and isolation, and take exercise in an environment where many others are suffering in similar ways, thereby improving quality of life and decreasing pain and disability. Simple advice such as the wearing of supportive cushioned trainers on the feet may make an enormous difference to daily walking.

Box 3.2 Non-drug therapies for osteoarthritis

- Education about the condition and its management for patients, relatives and carers
- A positive attitude and information about the fact that most people with osteoarthritis improve with time rather than deteriorate, as they learn to manage better
- Self-management programmes and contact with patient support organisations
- Social support by personal or telephone contact with other sufferers, volunteers, care-givers and professionals
- Weight reduction if the patient is overweight
- Aerobic exercise programmes
- Personalised exercise programmes in a warm environment, such as those at health or leisure clubs

---

- Range of movement (flexibility) physical therapy
- Muscle-strengthening exercises
- Walking aids
- Modified footwear and other orthotic devices (e.g. insoles or braces)
- Patellar taping
- Modification of activities to protect joints
- Aids to daily living
- Acupuncture
- Electrotherapy

The Western Ontario and McMaster Osteoarthritis Index (WOMAC) is a validated instrument for measuring disease-specific outcomes, and it is sensitive to change.[28] *Clinical Evidence* (Issue 5)[15] found one systematic review from 1997 that identified 11 randomised controlled trials (RCTs) of exercise in patients with osteoarthritis of the knee or hip. The review concluded that exercise regimes were beneficial but that 'more evidence was needed'. One study looked at the effects of a structured exercise programme on self-reported disability. The participants, who all had knee osteoarthritis, were randomised to one of three programmes, namely an aerobic exercise programme, a resistance exercise programme or a health education programme. The two exercise groups did better than the education group and showed significant but modest reductions in disability and pain. *Clinical Evidence*[15] also reported one systematic review from 1993 and three subsequent RCTs, and concluded that there was limited evidence to suggest that both exercise and education reduce pain and disability in patients with knee or hip osteoarthritis.

Physiotherapists can help patients to carry out suitable exercise for the affected joints, and target wasted or weak muscles for therapy. They often have leaflets available that patients can take home with them to remind them what they should do on a regular basis. Although good evidence has yet to be provided by well-designed studies, patients and therapists often use bipolar electrotherapy and pulsed ultrasound with good results in individuals. The experience of being assessed, listened to and taught by a knowledgeable professional for longer than the average medical or nursing consultation may have added benefits for patients who are struggling with disability, pain and frustration.

An occupational therapist can make an assessment of how well the patient is managing everyday activities. Modifying the way in which tasks are done, or providing aids, can make all the difference to a patient

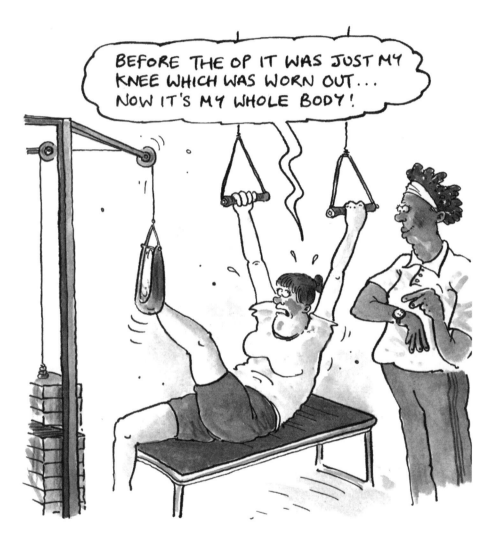

who is frustrated by being unable to perform the activities that he or she did without thinking before the pain, stiffness and disability developed.

Mr J had always been a keen gardener in the small back garden of his terraced house on a steep hill. Now he could only manage the steps and kneel to weed with difficulty, and his hands would not grip the tools. The occupational therapist was able to show him some tools that he could use and discuss with him the provision of rails to help him up and down the steps. He began to redesign the garden so that he could manage it more easily within his disabilities and have fresh hope that he would be able to do more himself, and not rely on his daughter to do it all. Despite his pain and disability, he was much more cheerful.

Discuss diet and complementary therapies. Patients will try them out anyway, and you need to know what they are trying as part of the management plan. Weight reduction is helpful for reducing pain and increasing function. A high vitamin C intake has been associated with a reduction in the progression of osteoarthritis of the knee,[29] and lower vitamin D concentrations with faster progression of knee and hip osteoarthritis, but as yet there is no evidence of any benefit from vitamin supplements. Chondroitin and glucosamine have been shown to be of benefit at least in the short term, and the absence of side-effects makes them a popular choice for many patients.[29] Several studies have shown an improvement in symptoms as a result of the use of acupuncture.[3,26]

Drug therapies

Box 3.3 lists the main drug treatments for pain relief.

Drug therapies for osteoarthritis should be used with caution, as many sufferers will have risk factors that affect the choice of medication. Non-steroidal anti-inflammatory drugs (NSAIDs) are probably over-used. When they have been started because of severe pain and signs of inflammation, re-evaluate as soon as the pain and inflammation are under control, so that the patient can be switched to simple analgesics as soon as possible. Systematic reviews of RCTs have shown that simple analgesics and NSAIDs produce short-term relief of pain in osteoarthritis, although there is no *clear* evidence of the superiority of

NSAIDs (but listen to the individual patient – it is not your pain!). One study compared two doses of ibuprofen with paracetamol and found no differences between the three groups.

When an NSAID is needed, the current evidence[30,31] does not favour any one of these drugs above another. Most trials were poorly designed and short term. Consider safety, patient acceptability and cost when making your choice. Look also at the information in Chapter 4 on NSAIDs.

Box 3.3 Drug treatment for osteoarthritis – stepping up from 1 to 3

1 Adequate doses of simple analgesics (e.g. paracetamol)
2 Topical preparations (e.g. NSAIDs, rubefacients, capsaicin)
3 NSAIDs (only if symptoms are not controlled by other means or during acute flare-up; step down after control has been obtained)
4 Intra-articular corticosteroid injection (for acute flare-up or if the patient is unfit for surgery)
5 Intra-articular hyaluronan injections (an expensive option that is now available for patients who are unfit for surgery)

Clinical Evidence[15] looked at the effects of topical agents in osteoarthritis. These are frequently used, but there is no *good* evidence to demonstrate that they are superior to simple rubefacients. A systematic review from 1996 identified 86 trials comparing topically applied NSAIDs with placebo. These agents were generally found to be more effective than placebo. One of the studies included in the review compared topical piroxicam gel with oral ibuprofen, 1200 mg daily, and found no significant difference in the pain relief (good or excellent relief in 60% compared to 64% of cases).

Intra-articular injection of the knee

Systematic reviews of RCTs have not shown any clear evidence of benefit from intra-articular injection of various drugs (glucocorticoids or hyaluronan) compared with placebo.[15] In some RCTs both the placebo and the active ingredient groups showed substantial improvements relative to the baseline measurements. Simple aspiration of the knee joint may be just as effective – but the evidence for this is lacking.

Joint replacement surgery

Constant pain, particularly at rest or at night, is often the deciding factor with regard to joint replacement. Some surgeons follow the New Zealand criteria[32] (see Box 3.4) or a similar list when deciding at what stage to embark on joint replacement.

Box 3.4 New Zealand criteria: severity is scored out of a maximum possible value of 100; candidates for surgery score more than 45.

Pain:	severity 0–20	duration 0–20
Function:	walking difficulty 0–10	other 0–10
Joint damage:	pain on passive movement 0–10	other/X-ray 0–10
Other:	other joints 0–10	work, care giving, independence 0–10

Patients give more priority to the category 'other', and you might want to consider changing the balance in this list to give more points to functional impairment and fewer points to joint damage. Joint damage and the X-ray appearance often correlate poorly with the degree of pain and loss of function.

Hip replacement

One systematic review of RCTs and observational studies found that hip replacement is effective for at least 10 years. Uncontrolled observational studies suggest that hip replacement is effective for even longer-term periods.[15] Fatal pulmonary embolism occurs in 0.1– 0.2% of cases, and the overall death rate is 0.3–0.4%. Two reliable observational studies showed that the rate of revision was about 1% per year, but most revisions are not required until at least 10 years after operation.[15] Observational studies found that people over 75 years of age or younger than 45 years, and those who were obese, did less well and were less satisfied with the outcome after hip replacement.

Knee replacement

The studies on total knee replacement have tended to concentrate on the survival of the prosthesis rather than on patient outcomes, but two systematic reviews concluded that knee joint replacement is effective.[15]. Observational studies published since the systematic reviews did show that quality of life improved after all forms of knee replacement. The Medical Outcomes Study Short Form (SF36) was used for a cohort study of 52 patients aged 55–74 years who had knee replacements.[33] The scores for quality of life improved, but remained significantly below that for other individuals of the same age who were not affected by osteoarthritis. Similarly, in another study,[34] physical functioning and pain scores in men and pain, vitality, emotional and mental health scores in women all improved after knee joint replacement. Comparison with age-matched controls showed that their scores were still below those of their contemporaries even after the joint replacement. Patients will be on crutches for about three months after surgery, but are likely to be able to dispense with their walking stick (or use one instead of two) after full mobilisation. They will still need to avoid vigorous sports such as tennis or skiing. Death rates are low, and are quoted as 0.63% for the first 30 days following admission for knee replacement, with a 24% risk of a deep vein thrombosis. Revision appears to be the main problem, with higher rates than for hip replacement, namely 3.8% over 4.1 years for tricompartment prostheses, 9.2% over 4.6 years for unicompartment prostheses, and 7.2% over 3.6 years for bicompartment prostheses. Aseptic loosening causes the majority of revisions, and the balance of benefit to harm is about the same as for hip replacements.[15]

However, many people with osteoarthritis are elderly and often have several other health problems that need to be taken into consideration when contemplating surgical intervention. Surgery may need to be performed under epidural anaesthesia, but age alone should not be a bar to joint replacement, as the latter significantly improves quality of life and reduces the need for pain relief with all its attendant risks.

Reflection exercises

Exercise 6

As a practice nurse/receptionist/practice manager/physiotherapist/ community pharmacist/doctor/any other member of the team caring for patients with osteoarthritis, you might audit the proportion of those patients with osteoarthritis who have been given adequate advice and help with non-drug therapies. Draw up a list of patients with osteoarthritis from your disease register (manual or computer generated). If you are not confident about how to do an audit, consult reference books such as *Making Sense of Audit*,[35] or ask for help from your education lead (or audit group, if you have one in your primary care organisation).

If you do not have a disease register, now might be the time to set one up, searching on medication and recorded diagnosis, and planning how to keep it up to date with a designated disease code entry.

Use a check-list (e.g. the one shown in Box 3.2) to design a short questionnaire, or base it on the one below. Set a standard for your audit (e.g. 80% have answered 'yes' to 10 out of 14 of the questions).

Example of a questionnaire for patients

Please put a tick to show whether you have discussed the following issues about your osteoarthritis with the health professionals you have seen:

	Yes	No	I would like more information
Information about osteoarthritis			
What medical treatments are available			
How to manage your condition yourself			
What voluntary organisations are available			
What support and help are available			
What sports and leisure facilities would help			
Whether weight loss would help			
Whether exercise would help			
Flexibility exercises			
Muscle-strengthening exercises			
Walking aids (e.g. sticks)			
Special footwear			
What activities to avoid			
What gadgets or adaptations to your home would help you with everyday life			

Decide how the patient can complete the answers. Do you want to mail out the form so that you obtain answers from those patients who do not attend the surgery, or are you going to start by tackling just those patients who come into the surgery, pharmacy or physiotherapy department? Some patients may need help with reading or writing, either because of literacy problems, or because their English is not good. You may want to involve all of the reception staff at an early stage if you are going to ask for their help. Decide whether:

- you are going to ask every patient with osteoarthritis in the next 4 weeks by flagging their medical records in some way
- you are going to use the computer to select patients randomly (this is particularly useful if you are going to mail patients).

Plan how you can increase the number of patients who have adequate non-drug management – perhaps by increasing the expertise of a couple of the staff (possibly the practice nurse and physiotherapist) to provide a resource for all of the practice. You might wish to involve patients who have a positive attitude towards their condition to provide support and advice, or utilise the local group of a voluntary society where one is available (or alternatively help to set one up).

You or another practice team member could help to set up a walking club with volunteers from the community, or ask members of a local walking club to start a rolling programme to build up the distances that patients could walk. In some areas the parish council has helped with such schemes, while in others the local ramblers club or the health promotion department have been involved.

Give feedback to the patients and staff who have helped with the audit about both what action is proposed, and what has been achieved at the completion of the action plan. Plan to repeat the audit (perhaps in 12 months) on completion of your action plan.

Exercise 7

As a doctor/medical secretary/physiotherapist, you might discuss informally with other doctors/physiotherapists the criteria that they use for referral for consideration of surgery or physiotherapy. This would make explicit the reasons for referral.

You could show them the New Zealand scoring system[32] and modify it to be more patient-centred. Then obtain their agreement to provide your orthopaedic surgical colleagues with a structured referral letter containing your criteria and any contra-indications to surgery. Together the doctors and physiotherapists could draw up a set of criteria for referral for physiotherapy. Then the person who makes the referrals could use the criteria in a clear way so that everyone understands why the referral has been made. Remember to build in a way of evaluating the usefulness of the criteria at intervals and on completion of your action plan (e.g. you could take all the referrals for one month and check them against the criteria).

Now that you have completed one or more of the interactive reflection exercises in this chapter, transfer the information from this needs assessment to the empty templates. Use the personal development plan on pages 123–132 if you are working on your own learning plan, or the practice personal and professional development plan on pages 147–153 if you are working on a practice team learning plan. The conclusions reached at the end of each exercise will feature in the action plan. Don't forget to keep the evidence of your learning in your personal portfolio.

CHAPTER 4

Gout

What is gout?

Gout is an inflammatory joint disease caused by the deposition of crystals of the sodium salt of uric acid in the joints. The joints most commonly affected are the first metatarso-phalangeal joint, the mid-tarsal joints and the knee. It has a prevalence of about 1% of the population, and is most common in men (male : female ratio 5 : 1) aged 40–50 years.[36]

Gout cannot occur without hyperuricaemia (serum uric acid levels that are persistently higher than 0.4 mmol/L). Hyperuricaemia is very common, and is almost always due to inability of the kidney to excrete enough uric acid into the urine. This is usually due to genetic factors, although drugs (particularly diuretics) can also reduce renal excretion of uric acid. Alcohol and obesity can contribute to hyperuricaemia, but other dietary factors are of little importance. In some (but not all) people with high serum levels of uric acid, crystals grow preferentially in the cartilage and synovium of joints. They can then be shed into the joint space where they set up an acute, severe inflammatory synovitis that is self-limiting. If uric acid levels remain very high for a long period, deposits can form elsewhere (including subcutaneous tissues), forming characteristic 'tophi' that can lead to the destruction of the adjacent tissues, including the joints.

Diagnosis and clinical features

The typical acute attack is very characteristic. It usually starts at night, and may be precipitated by trauma or another illness. It affects one joint, quickly becomes excruciatingly painful, and the affected joint is hot and red. Attacks usually subside on their own within a few days, but the severity of the pain generally requires treatment to ease symptoms and hasten resolution. Occasionally attacks are polyarticular.

Gout with tophi is now uncommon, and rarely occurs in the absence of a history of preceding acute attacks. However, it can cause confusion as the deposits may mimic rheumatoid nodules. Atypical gout can occur in older women (generally those on diuretics and with compromised renal function) in whom tophi form on the fingers and elsewhere in the absence of any acute attacks.

In the typical middle-aged man there are usually a number of important associations with gout (see Box 4.1). When investigating a patient with gout, as much attention should be paid to associated cardiovascular risk factors as to the gout itself.

Gout is very rare in men under 25 years of age and in premenopausal women. If gout does occur in such groups they should be referred to specialists, as they may have an uncommon inborn error of metabolism that requires careful management and genetic counselling.

Box 4.1 Typical associations with gout in middle-aged men

A family history of gout
Obesity*
High alcohol intake*
Hypertension
Hypertriglyceridaemia
A family history of cardiovascular disease

* Factors that contribute directly to the hyperuricaemia.

Investigations

During the acute attack, no investigations should be undertaken other than possible aspiration of synovial fluid for crystal identification and to exclude sepsis if there is diagnostic uncertainty. Uric acid levels are often normal (and therefore misleading) during the acute attack.

During the intercritical phase (after the attack has subsided), check the uric acid level and renal function, and measure lipid levels and the blood pressure. Many men only have one or two attacks in a lifetime, but others will have more persistent trouble (on average, around two to four attacks each year). Annual review of blood pressure and renal function is recommended in those with persistent attacks or those on therapy for gout. Other investigations, including radiographs, are unhelpful.

Management

Management can be divided into four categories.[37,38]

The *acute attack* should be managed with anti-inflammatory medication, typically a 'decrescendo' regime of an NSAID (a large initial loading dose, high doses in the first 24–48 hours, and then quickly tailing off to nothing as the attack subsides). If NSAIDs are contra-indicated, a single high dose of steroid (around 40 mg) administered orally or intramuscularly is usually effective. So long as infection is absent, it is also safe to inject steroid into a gouty joint in order to treat the persistent inflammation which sometimes occurs. As in other situations, it is wise to limit steroid joint injections to a maximum of about four a year.

Recurrent acute attacks can be treated in one of two ways:

1　provision of a supply of an NSAID so that the patient can start the decrescendo regime as soon as they feel the attack coming on, or
2　low-dose regular treatment with colchicine (0.5 mg twice daily), which is an effective prophylactic so long as it is taken every day.

Control of hyperuricaemia is generally unnecessary. Reduce the levels of uric acid in:

- cases of gout with tophi
- patients in whom the acute attacks are very frequent and severe despite treatment
- patients in whom renal function is abnormal (persistently raised urea or creatinine levels).

Management of obesity, reduction of alcohol intake and the stopping of any drugs (e.g. salicylates or diuretics) that might be contributing to hyperuricaemia is often sufficient. If uric acid-lowering drugs are needed, then allopurinol is the drug of choice, but once started this needs to be a lifetime treatment. The doses that are required to keep uric acid levels low enough to prevent gout (more than 0.4 mmol/L) range from 100 to 800 mg/day. During the first few months of treatment more acute attacks are precipitated, so give concurrent low-dose colchicine or a regular NSAID. Uric acid-lowering drugs are over-used, and although they are relatively safe they can cause problems.

The decision to start treatment with such a drug should be a shared one after consideration of the other options. Many individuals opt to put up with and treat intermittent attacks rather than take lifetime drugs.

Asymptomatic hyperuricaemia should not be treated unless there is renal disease or serum levels are consistently very high (more than 0.7 mmol/L).

Common pitfalls in the diagnosis and management of gout

Most gout is easy to diagnose and manage. However, mistakes are common.[37] They include the following.

- Diagnosis of people with joint pain and mild hyperuricaemia as having gout. Most hyperuricaemic individuals do *not* get gout.
- Dismissal of gout because serum uric acid levels are normal during the acute attack.
- Misdiagnosis of septic arthritis. Septic arthritis and pseudogout are the two main differential diagnoses of acute severe attacks of arthritis in a single joint. The management of acute pseudogout is identical to that of acute gout, so it does not matter if the diagnosis is missed. However, if sepsis is missed the consequences can be fatal, so if there is any doubt aspirate synovial fluid for urgent bacteriological examination.
- Treatment of the acute attack with allopurinol or another hypo-uricaemic drug. This is disastrous, as it can precipitate terrible polyarticular attacks.
- Use of hypouricaemic therapy in the absence of confirmation of gout, and use of too high a dose of allopurinol in older patients with renal impairment. In both cases severe side-effects can occur.

Most gout can and should be managed in the community. However, given the above considerations, possible reasons for referral to a rheumatologist might include diagnostic uncertainty, severe uncontrolled or persistent acute attacks despite anti-inflammatory therapy, gout with tophi, and gout in atypical groups (men under 25 years of age and women under 45 years). You should be alert for serious renal or cardiovascular disease in these patients, and if this develops you might want to refer the patient to a nephrologist or cardiologist.

Reflection exercises

Exercise 8

As a GP, you could look at how well your treatment of gout compares with the best practice described in this chapter. If your practice is well computerised you should be able to run an audit to identify patients with gout. If not, search on your computer to find out which patients are taking allopurinol or colchicine. Alternatively, ask the receptionists to note down the names of the next 10 consecutive patients who request repeat prescriptions of allopurinol or colchicine. Select 10 of these patients with gout at random.

Look at the case notes of the 10 patients.

1 Have they had their lipid levels measured and renal function checked within the previous 12 months? (This should have been done.) If these test results are abnormal, check whether appropriate clinical action has been taken, e.g. patient started on statins or referred to a consultant physician.
2 Has a gouty joint been X-rayed during the previous three years? (This should not have been done to investigate gout.)
3 Have any gout-precipitating drugs such as diuretics or salicylates been discontinued and other appropriate medication satisfactorily substituted?

From the results of this audit decide whether anything has arisen to indicate that you or your GP colleagues need to learn more about gout or changing your practice.

Exercise 9

As a GP or practice nurse, you could look out all of the patient literature you have in your practice for people with gout and other musculoskeletal problems. Do you have any literature about musculo-skeletal conditions and how people can look after themselves and minimise any disability or loss of function? Does the literature match the most up-to-date thinking about best practice in clinical management? Or does it promote out-of-date practices and approaches, or use old terminology?

Choose gout and at least three other topics that are addressed in this book to do this exercise. You yourself need to be clear what the most up-to-date recommendations are in order to be able to check your literature and complete this exercise. If you do not have any suitable literature, what about drawing up your own leaflets in simple language to photocopy for patients?

Now that you have completed one or more of the interactive reflection exercises in this chapter, transfer the information from this needs assessment to the empty templates. Use the personal development plan on pages 123–132 if you are working on your own learning plan, or the practice personal and professional development plan on pages 147–153 if you are working on a practice team learning plan. The conclusions reached at the end of each exercise will feature in the action plan. Don't forget to keep the evidence of your learning in your personal portfolio.

CHAPTER 5

Non-steroidal anti-inflammatory drugs

How they work

Non-steroidal anti-inflammatory drugs (NSAIDs) reduce pain and inflammation and inhibit platelet aggregation. They are widely used, but do not appear to have any effect in reducing the disease process of the various types of arthritis – that is, they suppress the symptoms but do not prevent the progression of the disease. The drugs inhibit cyclo-oxygenase (COX), the enzyme that converts arachidonic acid into prostaglandins. The lowering of the prostaglandin levels is responsible for the pain relief and reduction in inflammation, but also causes the side-effects. Prostaglandins also protect the intestinal mucosa and maintain renal blood flow. COX-1 produces the prostaglandins that mediate gastric protection and renal perfusion and reduce platelet aggregation. COX-2 produces the prostaglandins that mediate the inflammatory response. Differences in the way that each NSAID inhibits the two enzymes COX-1 and COX-2 may explain why some of these drugs are more likely to cause side-effects than others. However, preferential COX-2 inhibitors (e.g. etodolac and meloxicam) and selective COX-2 inhibitors (e.g. rofecoxib and celecoxib) still have associated risks of gastrointestinal side-effects and are contraindicated in people with a history of peptic ulcer, perforation or bleeding. They may also have other long-term risks, and reports about the effects on the cardiovascular system with longer-term use are beginning to appear. A more balanced appraisal of the role of COX-2 inhibitors will have to wait for researchers to finish longer-term studies.

Do some work better than others?

Studies examining patient preferences for particular NSAIDs have not been replicated.[15] It seems likely that variations in patient preferences are either due to natural variations in disease activity or due to chance. Health professionals who are in daily contact with patients frequently encounter individuals who swear by a particular drug – but over the years find the same patients returning with the comment that they need a change.

> Dr D had almost given up trying to persuade Mrs N to change from acemetacin. She had joined the practice while already receiving repeats of the drug for her attacks of wrist tendinitis. Dr D had tried pointing out that her job as a data-entry clerk was related to her attacks and that there were safer ways of relieving her symptoms, but she just attended more often until he relented. Then her workload suddenly increased when her workmate left and she had a really bad flare-up. She returned to Dr D saying that she must have 'got used to the capsules' and could she have something stronger?

The only meta-analysis that found one drug to be better than another was funded by the manufacturer. The studies that it included were small, and a meta-analysis is merely a statistical procedure for combining the results of several studies. A meta-analysis cannot correct for flaws in the original studies, or variations in the quality or methods of the studies that it combines. A large RCT did not replicate the results.[15]

Risks associated with the use of NSAIDs

Gastrointestinal problems

A useful summary of current evidence about NSAIDs appeared in *Bandolier* in 1998.[39] Surveys have shown that many prescribers were unaware of the adverse events associated with NSAIDs. Between 1% and 3% of those using NSAIDs for a year develop gastrointestinal

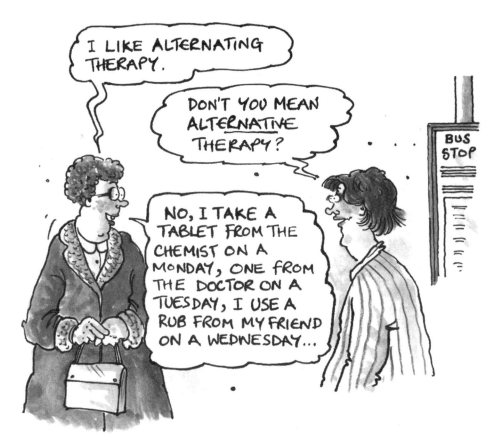

bleeding. Risk factors for serious gastrointestinal complications of NSAIDs include the following:

- a history of peptic ulcer or previous gastrointestinal bleeding
- age 75 years or over
- a history of heart disease
- smoking
- alcohol.

Women seem to be at higher risk than men. Without risk factors the 1-year risk of this adverse effect was quoted in this summary as being 0.08% (i.e. 8 in every 100 users of NSAIDs).

Some NSAIDs are more likely to cause problems than others. Ibuprofen is normally quoted as the baseline with which the other drugs are compared. Aspirin and diclofenac come near the bottom of the relative risks quoted (i.e. giving the least increased risk of gastrointestinal problems). Naproxen and indometacin are around the middle, and piroxicam, ketoprofen and especially azapropazone are the riskiest of the NSAIDs. It makes sense to use the least risky drug first, but in adequate dosage to relieve pain and swelling. Although the variation in efficacy between the different NSAIDs seems to be slight, the adverse effects differ considerably. Ibuprofen was found to be significantly less toxic than other NSAIDs when a meta-analysis of a combination of several studies was performed.[15]

In this meta-analysis the effect of increasing doses showed a linear relationship with increased adverse effects. Other systematic reviews have shown that the usual recommended doses were close to the ceiling effect, and that increasing the dose was no more effective in relieving pain or inflammation.

Always check before prescribing whether the patient is already using over-the-counter oral or topical NSAIDs. There is no point in adding naproxen to their ibuprofen (e.g. Brufen) or ibuprofen to their aspirin (e.g. Anadin or Aspros), and it does increase the risks considerably.

Other risks

A systematic review of 38 placebo-controlled trials found that NSAIDs increased the mean diastolic blood pressure by 5.0 mmHg (95% CI 1.2–8.7 mmHg).[15] Adverse effects on renal and liver function are listed, as well as oedema, blood dyscrasias, tinnitus, skin rashes and a host of others listed individually for each drug. There are long lists of interactions with other medications.

How to minimise the risks

Clinical Evidence[15] found no evidence to show that NSAIDs were more effective than simple analgesics in the treatment of acute musculo-skeletal conditions. However, the clinical trials were reported to be of poor quality. That means that one cannot rely on the results to give accurate information on which to base one's treatment decisions. One review of 17 trials for shoulder pain was unable to reach any firm conclusions, while another review of 84 studies of ankle pain was unable to group the studies together because of differences in treatments. It seems to be common sense to avoid the use of NSAIDs if simple analgesia will be as effective in relieving pain, or to use the least toxic NSAID, namely ibuprofen at 400 mg three times a day, for acute conditions.

Similarly, in osteoarthritis, paracetamol has been found to have much the same effect as ibuprofen or naproxen, with less toxicity for *most* patients. However, remember that paracetamol can cause problems of its own. Patients may already be taking it – sometimes in branded preparations that they do not realise contain paracetamol (e.g. Alvedol, co-codamol) – and high doses can cause hepatic or renal failure. Paracetamol can also be a problem in those patients who may have poor liver or kidney function.

Bear in mind that it is not *your* pain – so check that relief is adequate, whatever you are using, and discuss the risks with the patient. They may decide that the risks are worth taking for the benefits they will obtain, or that they are not worth taking, so record the discussion and treatment decisions. Some patients decide that using a rubefacient, or possibly a topical NSAID, is a preferable option to all the risks of systemic medication.

It is sensible to become familiar with the adverse profiles of a few NSAIDs. Include the selected drugs on your preferred drug list or practice formulary. For example, if you include tiaprofenic acid on your preferred list, you need to be aware that urinary frequency, dysuria, cystitis and haematuria may occur with this drug. Aseptic meningitis has very rarely been reported with the use of ibuprofen. Sulindac may precipitate Stevens–Johnson syndrome (erythema multiforme with a variable rash, blisters in the mouth and other body openings, conjunctivitis and even corneal ulceration or perforation). Hypersensitivity rashes or asthma are possible with any of the NSAIDS. You are more likely to detect an adverse effect quickly, and discontinue the drug, if you are aware of the possibility that the clinical picture is likely to have an iatrogenic cause. If all members of the practice agree to use NSAIDs from a selected list, it will be much easier for all staff to be alert for possible adverse effects.

Patients at high risk of gastrointestinal problems should receive anti-ulcer treatments with their NSAIDs. Misoprostol, omeprazole and ranitidine taken regularly have all been found to work better than a placebo in randomly controlled trials. However, the H_2-receptor antagonists that reduce acid secretion (ranitidine, cimetidine, famotizine and nizatidine) were not as effective as omeprazole (one of the proton-pump inhibitors that reduce acid production and heal ulcers more quickly than H_2-blockers) or misoprostol (a prostaglandin analogue). Some recent trials[39] suggested that omeprazole may be most effective, but the studies were not strictly comparable with earlier trials. Misoprostol causes more adverse effects, mainly abdominal pain and diarrhoea. Misoprostol may cause vaginal bleeding and should only be taken by women in their reproductive years if they are also taking adequate contraceptive precautions.

The presence of *Helicobacter pylori* is known to be associated with the development of peptic ulceration, and eradicating this organism often enables patients to cease taking their anti-ulcer medication. A randomised trial of eradication of *Helicobacter pylori*[15] in patients who needed to take NSAIDs suggests that this would be useful for reducing the risk of peptic ulcers.

The more recently introduced selective cyclo-oxygenase-2 (COX-2) inhibitors have become available with the hope of reducing the unwanted effects of NSAIDs on the gastrointestinal tract. Rofecoxib and celecoxib are as effective as other NSAIDs, dyspepsia appears to occur as often, but the occurrence of ulcers as indicated by endoscopic examination was similar to that observed in an inert placebo medication.[39] Peripheral oedema, dizziness and skin rashes are adverse reactions that may still occur with the COX-2 inhibitors, as with other NSAIDs. These drugs are more expensive than most of the older NSAIDs. Although they are specifically indicated for the relief of symptoms in osteoarthritis, their use is limited by the presence in many sufferers of other medical conditions and interacting medications such as warfarin, ACE inhibitors, beta-blockers, diuretics and amitriptyline. Make sure that you check for the long list of interactions with existing medications, especially if you are using the newer drug celecoxib, which is licensed for use in rheumatoid arthritis as well as osteoarthritis. Celecoxib is contraindicated in patients with sulphonamide sensitivity, and in pregnancy. It is too early to base decisions about the use of COX-2 inhibitors on good evidence. Early reports of adverse effects on the cardiovascular system suggest that caution is necessary, and it may be prudent to avoid their prolonged use until the long-term risks are clearer.

Reflection exercise

Exercise 10

As practice team members, you might join together in significant event monitoring. One member could present an incident at a team meeting about a patient who has suffered an adverse effect from the use of NSAIDs. Compare the management by the practice team with a guideline such as that from the Primary Care Rheumatology Society[27] (*see* also useful addresses and websites in the Appendix) and decide how to minimise adverse effects in future.

Several reasons for an adverse event usually become apparent when the incident is examined constructively. One team member might want or be asked to draw up a preferred list of NSAIDs (to increase the use of the least harmful drugs) for discussion at another meeting, or discussions might promote better adherence to the previously negotiated practice formulary.

Other organisational aspects may become apparent that have more general applications. For example, you may decide to review the arrangements for repeat prescribing if NSAIDs have been continued as repeat medication with insufficient review. The team meeting may identify a failure to pass on messages or information about a patient, and put new procedures in place. You may discover a need for better structuring of patient record summaries, or for the summary to be placed more prominently, in order to ensure that previous history is taken into account when prescribing.

Now that you have completed the interactive reflection exercise in this chapter, transfer the information from this needs assessment to the empty templates. Use the personal development plan on pages 123–132 if you are working on your own learning plan, or the practice personal and professional development plan on pages 147–153 if you are working on a practice team learning plan. The conclusions reached at the end of each exercise will feature in the action plan. Don't forget to keep the evidence of your learning in your personal portfolio.

CHAPTER 6

Rheumatoid arthritis

Most health professionals in primary care will have little experience of new presentations of rheumatoid arthritis, so it is important that you suspect it and refer early to a specialist team. However, because it is a chronic disease you need to be involved in the continuing management and aware of the problems that may arise.

What is rheumatoid arthritis?

This autoimmune disorder typically involves many joints and often many other systems. Most patients have a fluctuating course that results in progressive joint destruction, deformity and disability. Inability or reduction of ability to do productive work causes economic loss to individuals and society. The disorder affects about 0.5% of the population.[40] An easily assimilated reference book for the practice library, such as the *ABC of Rheumatology*,[26] will help to remind you of the salient features. The prognosis after diagnosis is unpredictable. Some people experience flare-ups and remissions, while others suffer an unremitting progression. Over the years, articular deformities and functional impairment occur with structural damage to the joints. About half of those diagnosed will be disabled or unable to work after 10 years,[41] and the disease shortens life expectancy.[42]

Diagnosis and clinical features

The clinical management of rheumatoid arthritis can be divided into two main phases:

- the first few years of often severe joint inflammation and pain
- the problems caused by disability and impairment in damaged joints that are now less inflamed.

Initial diagnosis

You are likely to suspect rheumatoid arthritis if the patient presents with the 'red flags' (*see* Chapter 2) of symmetrical multiple inflamed small joints together with other system involvement. An insidious onset may cause you more problems.

- Patients may present with fatigue and joints that are stiff in the morning. They may feel quite unwell in a non-specific way, but with no signs of joint inflammation or pain. Women who present with these symptoms after childbirth may be misdiagnosed as suffering from postnatal depression, only to develop more classic signs later on.
- Palidromic joint pain – in which joint swelling occurs in a few joints and rapidly disappears (often before the patient can get an appointment!) – can precede the development of classical rheumatoid arthritis by several years.
- Occasionally rheumatoid arthritis can present in just one joint, when you may easily confuse it with gout, pseudogout or infection.
- Tendon sheaths often become inflamed, with the risk of rupture and serious dysfunction.
- If rheumatoid arthritis occurs in the neck joints, subluxation may compress the spinal cord so that symptoms may include paraesthesia, sudden deterioration in hand function, sensory loss, abnormal gait, incontinence or retention of urine.
- Refer any patient with undiagnosed episodic peripheral polyarthritis.

Extra-articular symptoms and signs

Rheumatoid nodules are commonest at sites of pressure, such as the extensor surface of the forearms. Vasculitis results from the deposition of immune complexes in the vessel wall of small and (occasionally) larger blood vessels. This can cause digital infarction or skin ulcers. Eye conditions that may accompany rheumatoid arthritis include episcleritis or scleritis. Dry eyes as part of Sjögren's syndrome may present as a late complication. Other neurological complications include peripheral nerves trapped by the swelling of the joints or peripheral neuropathy due to the disease or to medication.

Making a record of your evaluation of a patient with rheumatoid arthritis

You might wish to structure your recording so that it is easy to retrieve and monitor progress or deterioration. You might use a Likert scale to ask the patient to grade their symptoms from none to very severe (as shown in Box 6.1), or the patient or health professional could mark the severity of the symptoms along a linear scale.

Box 6.1 Evaluation of a patient with RA

Symptoms

Degree of joint pain	None	Slight	Moderate	Severe	Very severe
Fatigue	None	Slight	Moderate	Severe	Very severe
Limitation of function	None	Slight	Moderate	Severe	Very severe
Duration of morning stiffness (hours):					

Physical examination
Name joints inflamed:

Loss of movement	None	Slight	Moderate	Severe	Very severe
Extra-articular signs present:					

Investigations
ESR or C-reactive protein
Others as indicated for monitoring treatment (*see* Table 6.1)

The American College of Rheumatology[43] has established criteria for improvement to be used in clinical trials. You could use these to set and audit your own standards of care. The criteria specify a reduction of joint swelling and tenderness, and improvement in at least three of the following: pain, function, patient and physician global assessments, and acute-phase reactants such as ESR measurements.

Non-steroidal anti-inflammatory drugs (NSAIDs)

NSAIDs are extremely useful for reducing pain, swelling and inflammation in rheumatoid arthritis. A good response does *not* mean that the patient does not have the disease – only that the disease process is not severe at present. All patients should start on NSAIDs and be given pain relief while they are awaiting their appointment for evaluation for second-line disease-modifying drugs which should normally be started within three months of diagnosis.

Management of patients on disease-modifying anti-rheumatic drugs (DMARDs)

Active rheumatoid arthritis may result in irreversible joint damage even in the early months of the disease. Although NSAIDs (or steroids in severe disease) may improve symptoms, DMARDs have the potential to reduce or prevent joint damage. The Primary Care Rheumatology Society (see Appendix for a list of useful addresses) has produced guidelines[27] for early referral, and you could use these to audit your own standards. All DMARDs are relatively slow-acting, with delays of between one and six months before remission. About two-thirds of patients respond, but you cannot predict in advance which drug will work, so progress should be assessed at six months in order to determine whether the DMARD should be changed. Each DMARD has specific toxicity for which monitoring arrangements must be made and baseline tests should be performed to establish whether patients are suitable (e.g. for liver disease, alcohol abuse, and renal impairment or lung disease). These monitoring arrangements vary from one place to another. You may have a shared protocol, or the monitoring may take place either entirely in hospital (often run by a specialist nurse) or entirely in primary care. Table 6.1 shows an example of primary care guidelines[44] for monitoring.

Rheumatologists frequently select methotrexate. The recommended low weekly dosage used in rheumatoid arthritis minimises the toxic side-effects seen when this drug is used at higher doses in malignant disease treatment. It is more likely to succeed and continuation rates are better than with other DMARDs[45] (more than 50% at 3 years). The beneficial effects of cyclosporin in modifying the disease process in rheumatoid arthritis are probably outweighed by its severe toxicity. It is usually reserved for those with severe disease who do not respond to other DMARDs.

Leflunomide is a new drug that seems to be as effective as other

Table 6.1 Guidelines for monitoring DMARDs[44]

Drug	Maintenance dose	Toxicity	Tests
Hydroxychloroquine	200 mg twice daily	Rash (infrequent), diarrhoea, retinal toxicity (rare)	None unless symptoms are present
Sulfasalazine	1000 mg 2–3 times daily	Rash, myelosuppression (infrequent), gastrointestinal intolerance	FBC* and liver function tests weekly for 1 month, monthly for 5 months, then every 6 months
Methotrexate (toxic effects may be less with folic acid)	7.5–15 mg **per week**	Gastrointestinal symptoms, stomatitis, rash, alopecia, myelosuppression (infrequent), hepatotoxicity, pulmonary toxicity (rare but serious)	FBC* monthly, and liver function tests every 3 months
Injectable gold salts	25–50 mg IM every 2–4 weeks	Rash, stomatitis, myelosuppression, thrombocytopenia, proteinuria	FBC* and urinalysis weekly for 1 month, then monthly. If urine protein is ++, send midstream urine specimen. If midstream urine is negative or protein is + + +, stop and refer
Oral gold	3 mg 1–2 times daily	As above but less frequent, but diarrhoea is common	As above, but rarely used as it is less effective than injectable gold
Azathioprine	50–150 mg daily	Myelosuppression, hepatotoxicity (infrequent), early flu-like illness with fever, gastrointestinal symptoms, elevated liver function tests	FBC* and liver function tests weekly for 1 month, then monthly
D-penicillamine	250–750 mg daily after initial very gradual increase in dose	Rash, stomatitis, proteinuria, myelosuppression, autoimmune disease (rare but serious)	FBC* and urinalysis weekly for 2 months, then monthly

* FBC, full blood count.
Stop drug and refer if white blood cell count is < 3.0, platelets are < 120 or if liver function tests are deteriorating.

DMARDs. Three RCTs compared it with placebo and showed a reduction in disease activity.[15] Adverse reactions in the trial that compared it with methotrexate were very similar. Diarrhoea, nausea, alopecia and liver enzyme abnormalities were the most common adverse effects.

Newer therapies

Five RCTs have found that tumour necrosis factor (TNF) antagonists (etanercept and infliximab) reduce disease activity and joint inflammation. Short-term toxicity is low, but long-term effects have yet to be observed. Treatment regimes are still under trial. The main side-effect so far is an injection-site reaction. Other recorded effects include upper respiratory symptoms or infections, headache and diarrhoea. Antibodies to double-stranded DNA were found in 5–9% of the groups treated with etanercept and in 16% of those taking infliximab. Both drugs are administered by injection, but the effect on disease activity was seen within weeks rather than the period of months observed with traditional DMARDs.[15]

A cautionary tale

Press claims of a 'new cure for rheumatoid arthritis' (reported by many newspapers in November 2000) were, as usual, much exaggerated. Rituximab had been tested in a small-scale trial of 20 patients, and was used together with cyclophosphamide and prednisolone. Rituximab is already used in the treatment of lymphoma to destroy B-cells (the white blood cells that make antibodies). The theory is that, once destroyed, the new cells will not make the same mistake of producing the auto-antibodies that trigger rheumatoid arthritis.

It will be many years before we know whether this approach is useful, effective and safe. Many such stories that appear every year under seductive headlines bring hopeful patients to their doctor to ask for the 'new cure' that they have read about.

Oral corticosteroids

Systematic reviews of RCTs have shown benefit from short-term treatment in reducing disease activity and joint inflammation.

Longer-term treatment with low-dose corticosteroids (10 mg daily or less) may reduce damage to joints while treatment continues. However, long-term treatment, even at this low dose, is associated with the familiar adverse effects of corticosteroid use, namely hypertension, diabetes, osteoporosis, infections, gastrointestinal ulcers, obesity and hirsutism.

Other management issues

Practice teams will see few patients who present with the acute manifestations of rheumatoid arthritis, and much of the early management of the pain and inflammation will be achieved by early referral to the secondary care sector or by using shared protocols for that care once the diagnosis has been established.

The practice team will be more involved in the continuing management of the chronic remitting part of the illness.

People with chronic debilitating disease need support and a secure relationship with at least one or two health professionals. Patient preference will probably determine who those individuals are. The British League against Rheumatism (*see* list of useful addresses in the Appendix) have set out some standards for care for arthritis. For primary care these include the following.

1   The general practitioner should discuss the nature of arthritis and examine the joints at an early stage.
2   The general practitioner should explain the role of:

- exercise as a possible treatment
- physiotherapy as a possible treatment
- weight control
- footwear/chiropody as a possible treatment
- first-line NSAID treatment
- second-line DMARD treatment
- the purpose of referral and what might be expected from the rheumatology or orthopaedic department
- steroid injections
- oral steroids.

The role of the GP or practice nurse also includes monitoring the general health of the patient. All of those involved in the care of the patient should consider the prevention and treatment of osteoporosis, the systemic effects of rheumatoid arthritis and the adverse effects of medication. Be alert for depression, which can accompany any chronic illness, especially one that may cause social isolation through immobility. Other problems include loss of employment and low self-esteem because of the patient's inability to do what they used to do. You may want to add gastroprotective therapy, hormone replacement therapy, or bisphosphonates to their NSAID and DMARD.

Physiotherapists and occupational therapists can help with advice on alternative ways of carrying out tasks and on aids to mobility or daily living. If there is much loss of function, employment modification or social service intervention may also be needed.

Reflection exercises

Exercise 11

As a receptionist/practice manager/practice nurse/doctor/physiotherapist/others involved in the care of patients with rheumatoid arthritis, you might ask all affected patients about their care, as any one practice will not have many people with rheumatoid arthritis. Look at the exercise on osteoarthritis if you want to use a questionnaire. You could use a questionnaire along the lines of the following, but remember that many people with rheumatoid arthritis have difficulty in writing.

Example of how to set up your questionnaire

Please tick the answer nearest to what you think:

I feel I understand about:	Hardly anything	A little	A fair amount	Quite a lot	I am well informed
exercise as a possible treatment					
physiotherapy as a possible treatment					
the need for weight control					
non-steroidal anti-inflammatory medicines					
You could add other questions from the section on standards for care in general practice					

You might want to set up a focus group in which patients could discuss what they feel is good about their care and what could be improved. Think about how disabled patients could get to a central venue (could you use volunteer drivers?). You will need to set up some priming questions, so that the group discussion is partially structured. Ask for input on how the patients view their rheumatoid arthritis, what they know about the disease, and what other needs they have. Do they have a realistic picture of what adverse effects and benefits might be associated with the various interventions? Are they receiving all of the social and physical help that they need? What else is required and how could it be provided? For example, it might be possible to negotiate exercise sessions in a heated pool (either a children's warm learning pool or one in a health club) as a resource for the primary care organisation. You might get some innovative ideas that had not occurred to health staff!

Do not forget to give feedback to the patients who have helped in this exercise about what action is proposed and what has been achieved.

Exercise 12

If you are a practice manager/practice nurse/district nurse/phleboto-mist/ doctor/specialist nurse/receptionist with responsibility for mon-itoring repeat prescribing, you could select all of the patients on prescriptions for disease-modifying anti-rheumatic drugs. Examine the records to establish how many (if any) are receiving care under shared-care protocols. You might look at the paper describing how an audit was conducted elsewhere.[20]

If there are no shared-care protocols, present that information at a team meeting for considering setting up a small working group for introducing them.

If you have shared-care protocols for monitoring DMARDs, audit how well the standards for these are met by comparing what has been done with the standards set in the protocols (e.g. frequency of blood results, who looked at them, and the action taken). Report the results to the practice team so that any remedial action can be implemented or congratulations given. For example, you might find that the system is not working because of organisational changes (e.g. some housebound patients are now visited by a district nursing assistant instead of the district nurse, and the assistant is not trained to take blood), or that results are not received by the practice or secondary care clinic in time for their next review appointment.

Now that you have completed one or more of the interactive reflection exercises in this chapter, transfer the information from this needs assessment to the empty templates. Use the personal development plan on pages 123–132 if you are working on your own learning plan, or the practice personal and professional development plan on pages 147–153 if you are working on a practice team learning plan. The conclusions reached at the end of each exercise will feature in the action plan. Don't forget to keep the evidence of your learning in your personal portfolio.

CHAPTER 7

Systemic lupus erythematosus and similar connective tissue disorders

Systemic lupus erythematosus (SLE) is described in more detail than the other connective tissue disorders in order to provide an example of how such a condition might be managed. The connective tissue disorders have much in common and are often difficult to differentiate. Diagnosis is normally a secondary care function, but you need to know enough to detect that the patient needs this in the first place. The continuing management of the impairment caused by the condition is very much a part of the responsibilities of the primary care team.

What is systemic lupus erythematosus?

SLE is one of a group of interrelated and overlapping autoimmune rheumatic disorders. Lupus can affect the joints, muscles, skin, kidneys, nervous system, lungs, heart and blood cells. It affects women eight to ten times more frequently than men, and often first appears in women of childbearing years (18–45 years of age). Black women (African-American, Native American, Asian and Hispanic) are affected more often than Caucasian women. Lupus can also affect children, the elderly and men. It can affect more than one member of a family, but there have been no studies which demonstrate that it is an inherited disease. The prevalence of SLE is about 30 cases per 100 000 individuals. Although you are unlikely to encounter many patients with this condition, you need to be aware of the seriousness and complexity of SLE. The main obstacle to diagnosis is its rarity, as a result of which the diagnosis is not considered.[26]

Clinical features

Lupus is often difficult to diagnose because manifestations vary from one person to another and can fluctuate with time. Nearly all people with lupus experience changes in disease activity. Sometimes the disease may flare up, while at other times there may be remission and no evidence of lupus at all. Fever, weight loss and fatigue may be among the first signs of the illness. A skin rash may develop on the face, neck or arms, especially after exposure to the sun. This rash may involve the nose and cheeks and appear as a butterfly-shaped rash.

Painful swelling of the joints and prolonged stiffness in the morning may occur. The symptoms may mimic early rheumatoid arthritis. About 20% of patients develop deformity of the hands due to the fact that the tendons are affected. Inflammation of the surface of some organs (serositis), such as the heart and lungs, can cause painful breathing or shortness of breath. Ulcers (usually painless) may occur in the mouth or nose.

The kidneys can be affected without producing symptoms, although oedema of the legs may occur. Lupus affecting the kidneys may cause proteinuria, haematuria and high blood pressure. People with SLE may experience depression or difficulty in concentrating, either due to the disease itself or as a reaction to living with a chronic disease. Seizures may occur but are rare.

Diagnosis

The diagnosis of SLE is made from the clinical history, physical examination and test results. Tests that are commonly performed[24] include a blood count, assessment of kidney and liver function, urinalysis, antinuclear antibody (ANA) test, chest X-ray and electrocardiogram. The specialist, to whom you should refer the patient at an early stage, may recommend additional tests.

Management

Treatment of SLE depends on which organs are affected and the severity of their involvement. Because lupus may assume many different forms, finding the most effective treatment may take time.

Sunscreens with a sun protection factor (SPF) of at least 15 and protection from ultraviolet rays from the sun as well as avoidance of tanning beds are recommended even if the skin is not involved, as ultraviolet light can trigger a flare-up.

Aspirin or non-steroidal anti-inflammatory drugs (NSAIDs) may be recommended for joint manifestations. Antimalarial medications may be useful for treating skin and joint problems and serositis, and may prevent flare-ups of the disease.

Corticosteroids are frequently used and have transformed the outlook for patients with SLE. The dosage is dependent on the organs involved and the severity of their involvement. Much of the increased mortality in the later course of the disease is due to the side-effects of steroid use (weight gain, oedema, easy bruising, osteoporosis, hypertension, diabetes and increased risk of infection). Patients usually reduce the dosage of the steroid once a flare-up has settled, in order to minimise the adverse effects.

Immunosuppressive medications such as azathioprine and cyclophosphamide may be used to treat SLE, especially if the kidneys are involved. Other such medications of potential benefit include methotrexate, chlorambucil and cyclosporin. These may be used if corticosteroids are not effective, or in conjunction with a lower dose of corticosteroids (to reduce side-effects). These drugs may suppress bone marrow, and monitoring is required, often with a shared-care protocol between primary and secondary care (*see* section on monitoring in rheumatoid arthritis in Chapter 5), or by specialist nurses. The drugs may also increase the risk of infection and cancer. Sometimes the kidneys fail even with the use of corticosteroids and immunosuppressive drugs, and kidney dialysis may be necessary. If failure is permanent, a transplant may be considered.

Living with systemic lupus erythematosus

The diversity of SLE makes it a difficult condition to manage. Care may become fragmented between several specialists. The primary care team has an important role in supporting patients and co-ordinating treatment. Recognising when the symptoms are getting worse and knowing how to treat them can reduce the likelihood of permanent tissue or organ damage. Early treatment can also reduce the time spent on higher doses of medication. Advice on leading a healthy lifestyle and adopting a sensible exercise programme can reduce the risk of cardiovascular disease and help to slow bone loss. Appropriate exercises also increase flexibility and strengthen the muscles that help to stabilise the joints, as well as giving a psychological boost. Support groups can provide reassurance and help patients to feel more in control of the illness (see list of useful addresses in the Appendix). Patients may need advice from occupational physicians or employment advisers about suitable jobs or modifications to their present employment.

Other systemic connective tissue disorders

Brief accounts of three other significant systemic disorders are given below. Think about the implications in the same way as you have done for systemic lupus erythematosus.

Raynaud's phenomenon

- Raynaud's phenomenon is a common vasospastic disorder of the extremities, usually affecting the fingers, in which the digits go through a triphasic colour change consisting of pallor, cyanosis and hyperaemia.
- Raynaud's phenomenon is about four times more common in women than in men, and most cases are benign (primary).[37] A minority of cases are secondary to some other condition, including any systemic rheumatic disease (particularly systemic sclerosis), vibration injury, and chemical or drug exposure, e.g. to beta-blockers.
- Patients should be examined for signs of a systemic disease, such as telangiectasia or the tight skin over the fingers that is seen in systemic sclerosis. A high ESR (>25) or a positive antinuclear factor test also suggest secondary Raynaud's. All investigations are normal in primary Raynaud's phenomenon.
- Management depends on the frequency and severity of attacks. All sufferers should refrain from smoking and avoid local or general cold exposure. Calcium-channel blockers such as nifedipine can be helpful. Patients with severe Raynaud's phenomenon, or in whom a secondary cause is suspected, should be referred for a specialist opinion.

Sjögren's syndrome

- Sjögren's syndrome is the commonest form of autoimmune disease in the community. It occurs predominantly in women (female : male ratio 9 : 1), and is seen mainly in people in their forties or fifties.[37]
- It is characterised by a lymphocytic infiltration of exocrine glands (especially the parotid and lacrimal glands), leading to reduced secretion and hence dry eyes (which can lead to ulceration – keratoconjunctivitis sicca) and a dry mouth. Salivary gland enlargement, vaginal dryness, a mild polyarthritis and numerous other systemic features may occur.
- Sjögren's syndrome may occur in association with any systemic rheumatic disease (including rheumatoid arthritis) or on its own. In most cases it runs a slow and benign course, although occasionally lymphoma can develop.
- Most patients have a positive antinuclear factor test.
- The mainstay of therapy is to keep dry mucosal surfaces moist through local applications. Artificial tears are particularly important to help to minimise the risk of local ulceration. NSAIDs and antimalarial drugs may help to relieve the polyarthritis.

The seronegative spondarthritides

- The seronegative spondarthritides are a group of overlapping disorders associated with the HLA-B27 haplotype and common in young adults. The group includes ankylosing spondylitis, reactive arthritis and psoriatic arthritis. In each of these diseases a spinal arthritis, peripheral arthritis and/or enthesopathy (inflammation at the insertions of ligaments or tendons into bones, such as a plantar fasciitis or achilles tendinitis) may occur. A family history of one of the disorders is common.[37]
- *Ankylosing spondylitis* is common in young men, and usually presents with low backache and morning stiffness. Hallmarks of this condition include radiographic sacroiliitis and a good response to NSAIDs.
- *Reactive arthritis* is common in young adults (especially men) and is an arthropathy that develops 2 to 4 weeks after an infection of the genitourinary or gastrointestinal tracts. Skin and eye inflammation may accompany the lower limb, asymmetrical arthropathy and enthesopathy.

- *Psoriatic arthritis* is an inflammatory polyarthritis that occurs in patients with psoriasis, and a variety of different types of peripheral or spinal arthropathy may occur. The course is unpredictable, but it is generally benign.

You may want to look at one or more of these conditions in more detail, particularly if you have identified specific personal or practice learning needs.

Reflection exercise

Exercise 13

As a practice team, you might use significant incident analysis to examine the medical records of a patient with SLE. You will be able to learn some useful lessons about the difficulties of diagnosis and co-ordination of management between specialists. You might wish to introduce a shared-care patient record for these few patients so that they and all of the staff involved in their care are aware of each other's actions.

> Now that you have completed the interactive reflection exercise in this chapter, transfer the information from this needs assessment to the empty templates. Use the personal development plan on pages 123–132 if you are working on your own learning plan, or the practice personal and professional development plan on pages 147–153 if you are working on a practice team learning plan. The conclusions reached at the end of each exercise will feature in the action plan. Don't forget to keep the evidence of your learning in your personal portfolio.

CHAPTER 8

Polymyalgia rheumatica and giant-cell arteritis

What are they?

Most authorities now regard these two conditions as being very closely related. About 50% of patients with symptoms of giant-cell arteritis have symptoms and signs of polymyalgia rheumatica, and 15–50% of those with polymyalgia rheumatica have symptoms and signs of giant-cell arteritis. Giant-cell arteritis is also known as temporal or cranial arteritis.

Polymyalgia rheumatica is a rheumatic disorder that is associated with moderate to severe muscle pain and stiffness in the neck, shoulder and hip area. Stiffness is most noticeable in the morning. This disorder may develop rapidly – in some patients overnight. In other people, polymyalgia rheumatica develops more gradually. The cause of the disorder is not known. However, possibilities include immune system abnormalities and genetic factors. The fact that polymyalgia rheumatica is rare in people under the age of 50 years suggests that it may be linked to the ageing process.

Untreated giant-cell arteritis can lead to serious complications, including permanent loss of vision and stroke. *Patients must learn to recognise the signs of giant-cell arteritis, because they can develop them even after the symptoms of polymyalgia rheumatica have disappeared.* They need to know that they should report any symptoms that might herald giant-cell arteritis to the doctor immediately, and members of the practice team should all be aware of the urgency of the condition.

Clinical features

The primary symptoms of polymyalgia rheumatica are moderate to severe stiffness and muscle pain near the neck, shoulders or hips. The stiffness is more severe upon waking or after a period of inactivity, and typically lasts longer than 30 minutes. People with this condition may also have influenza-like symptoms, including fever, weakness and weight loss.

Early symptoms of giant-cell arteritis may also resemble those of influenza. As the condition progresses, the patient is likely to experience headaches, pain in the temples, and blurred or double vision. Pain may also affect the jaw and tongue.

Investigations

The erythrocyte sedimentation rate (ESR) is usually, but not always, very high. Patients may have a normocystic anaemia and raised hepatic enzymes, which together with the weight loss often suggests a hidden malignancy. Other investigations that have been suggested[26] are listed in Box 8.1.

Box 8.1 Suggested investigations for:

Polymyalgia rheumatica
- ESR
- Acute-phase proteins
- Full blood count
- Biochemical profile
- Protein electrophoresis
- Bence–Jones protein
- Thyroid function
- Chest X-ray
- Rheumatoid factor
- Muscle enzymes (if muscle weakness is present)

Giant-cell arteritis
- ESR
- C-reactive protein
- Full blood count
- Liver function tests
- Consider temporal artery biopsy, but do not delay treatment if it is not rapidly available

---

As can be seen from the long list above, the diagnosis is one of exclusion.

Management

Treatment with steroids is mandatory and urgent. Remember that patients with polymyalgia rheumatica may develop giant-cell arteritis quite suddenly.

Patients with polymyalgia rheumatica should be 80% better within 5 days. Local recommendations vary, but a commonly suggested scheme of treatment with prednisolone for polymyalgia rheumatica[44] is as follows:

* 15 mg/day for 4 weeks
* then 12.5 mg/day for 4 weeks
* then 10 mg/day for 4 weeks
* then reduce by 1 mg/month.

Around 50% of patients with polymyalgia rheumatica can discontinue therapy within 2 years, but recurrences are most frequent during the first 18 months. The ESR may not be raised in recurrences, so treat symptomatically.

Azathioprine can be used for its steroid-sparing effect (50–75 mg/day). Non-steroid anti-inflammatory drugs are useful while reducing steroids.

Patients with visual symptoms of giant-cell arteritis may need 40–80 mg of prednisolone daily urgently at the onset of the disease, reducing by 5 mg every 3–4 weeks until they are on 10 mg/day, and then reducing as suggested for polymyalgia rheumatica above.

Remember the potential adverse effects of corticosteroids and the requirement for prevention of osteoporosis (*see* Chapter 9).

Reflection exercise

Exercise 14

As a practice manager/nurse/clinical governance lead/audit receptionist/doctor, you might audit the records of patients with a diagnosis of polymyalgia rheumatica and giant-cell arteritis to establish whether the practice guidelines for reducing oral steroids are being followed. It should be relatively easy to check medication records in a practice with computerised records, but paper records will need manual searching. You could also check for adherence to recommended treatment by looking at the frequency with which medication is requested. Discuss the results with all of the staff involved. You could take appropriate action to add prompts to medication if patients are not being reviewed or managed in the agreed way. Re-audit after your action and feed back the results to all of those involved.

Now that you have completed the interactive reflection exercise in this chapter, transfer the information from this needs assessment to the empty templates. Use the personal development plan on pages 123–132 if you are working on your own learning plan, or the practice personal and professional development plan on pages 147–153 if you are working on a practice team learning plan. The conclusions reached at the end of each exercise will feature in the action plan. Don't forget to keep evidence of your learning in your personal portfolio.

CHAPTER 9

Osteoporosis

What is osteoporosis?

Osteoporosis is a reduction in bone mass and density that leads to increased risks of fracture, back pain and curvature of the spine.

The main consequence of osteoporosis is the increased tendency to fracture with minor trauma (fragility fractures) and the subsequent loss of function and quality of life. Colles' fracture affects 15% of women and vertebral fractures affect up to 20% (although many cases are asymptomatic). Hip fracture affects one in four women who live to 85 years, of whom 25% die within 12 months and more than 50% remain disabled.[26] The incidence of osteoporotic fracture is increasing more than would be expected solely as a result of the increasing age of the population, so attention to risk factors (*see* Boxes 9.1 and 9.2) might prevent some of these cases.

Box 9.1 Risk factors for osteoporosis

- Female
- Elderly
- Early menopause
- Smoking
- High alcohol intake
- Physical inactivity
- Thin body type
- Heredity
- Other causes of secondary osteoporosis (*see* Box 9.2)

Box 9.2 Types of osteoporosis

Primary
- Type 1 (postmenopausal)
- Type 2 (age-related bone loss)
- Idiopathic (at ages less than 50 years)

Secondary
- Endocrine (thyrotoxicosis, primary hyperparathyroidism, Cushing's syndrome, hypogonadism from anorexia nervosa or excessive exercise)
- Gastrointestinal (malabsorption, e.g. due to coeliac disease, partial gastrectomy, liver disease)
- Rheumatological (rheumatoid arthritis, ankylosing spondylitis)
- Malignancy (multiple myeloma, metastases)
- Corticosteroids

Who should you investigate?

Currently there is no rationale for population screening for low bone density with dual-energy X-ray absorptiometry (DEXA) scanning. It makes sense to target those who are most likely to be at risk from the above lists. You might investigate a perimenopausal woman who has risk factors, to help her to make a decision about using hormone replacement therapy. Similarly, you might wish to screen younger women with risk factors such as premature menopause due to an oophorectomy, or with anorexia nervosa. Other indications would be those patients with diseases that cause secondary osteoporosis (*see* Box 9.2), patients on more than 7.5 mg prednisolone daily or the equivalent for more than 6 months, or those with a fragility fracture. Only embark on screening if you are willing and able to make serial measurements of bone density to measure the rate of change. DEXA scan results are usually reported as T-scores (comparison with the young adult mean) and sometimes also as Z-scores (comparison with reference values for the same age). A simple classification of DEXA scan results is given in Table 9.1.

Table 9.1 DEXA scan results

	T score	*Fracture risk*	*Action*
Normal	>−1.0	Low	Lifestyle advice
Low bone mass (osteopenia)	−1.0 to −2.5	Medium	Lifestyle advice, investigate and treat
Osteoporosis	<−2.5	High	Lifestyle advice, investigate and treat

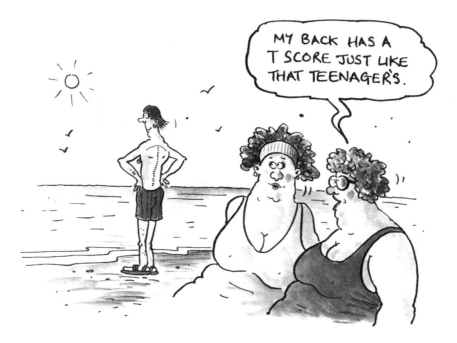

If low bone mass or osteoporosis is found, you should screen for underlying causes with the following investigations:

- serum calcium, phosphate, alkaline phosphatase and creatinine
- serum protein electrophoresis
- thyroid function tests
- serum testosterone in men
- urinary Bence–Jones protein, or 24-hour urinary calcium or creatinine excretion as indicated by the clinical findings and consultation with the laboratory.

Treatment for patients with osteopenia or osteoporosis

You will need to ensure that all patients who are at risk receive lifestyle advice (i.e. regular weight-bearing exercise, adequate nutrition including calcium and vitamin D, and avoidance of smoking or excess alcohol intake). Prevention of falls minimises fracture risk, and a useful summary of strategies appears in the *Drug and Therapeutics Bulletin* on managing falls in older people.[46] You will want to minimise other risk factors, but this may not be possible (e.g. in patients) who require oral steroid treatment. Education about osteoporosis for patients, carers and relatives is very helpful and the National Osteoporosis Society[47] (*see* list of useful addresses in the Appendix) produces relevant material as well as a patient helpline. The National Osteoporosis Society has produced useful guidelines for the prevention and management of corticosteroid-induced osteoporosis,[27] and you might use these to evaluate your own standards of care.

Pain relief is mainly achieved by analgesic medication working up from paracetamol in full dosage to opiates. Remember that opiates or opiate-like drugs may increase the risk of falling. Low-dose antidepressants are useful for their pain-modulating effects, and you might wish to refer patients whose pain is not adequately controlled to a pain clinic. Lumbar supports, transcutaneous nerve stimulators or acupuncture are useful in some patients.

Drug treatments for improving bone mass (or preventing further loss of bone mass) are summarised in the guidelines from the Royal College of Physicians,[18] and you could consider the medications in Table 9.2 for established osteoporosis or for osteopenia with a history of previous fracture.[48]

Table 9.2 Drugs to improve bone mass[3,26,48,49]

Vitamin D and calcium	Recommended daily dose is 800 IU of vitamin D and 0.5–1 g of calcium. This has been shown to reduce hip fracture in the frail elderly, and to produce a modest reduction in non-vertebral fracture in men and women over 65 years of age. Usually used as an adjunct to other treatments
Calcium	At 1000 mg daily has a less marked effect
Bisphosphonates	Poor absorption means that these drugs should be taken on an empty stomach, but they can cause gastrointestinal problems
Hormone replacement therapy	Treatment should be for at least 5 years to decrease the fracture risk, and long-term treatment risks (e.g. increased risk of cancer of the breast or prostate) must be balanced against gains
SERMS	Selective Estrogen Receptor Modulators such as raloxifene are useful for those women who do not require relief of hot flushes, or who need to avoid the oestrogen-stimulating effect on the endometrium or breast
Calcitonin	Available as a subcutaneous injection. It also has analgesic effects that are useful in acute fracture
Anabolic steroids	Androgenic side-effects make these unsuitable for women

A clear explanation of the way in which these drugs work and the need for long-term treatment helps patients to overcome their natural resistance to continuing to take medication when they cannot feel any immediate benefit from it.

Reflection exercises

Exercise 15

If you are a practice nurse/doctor/receptionist or secretary with audit responsibilities/community pharmacist, you might use a search strategy to identify patients who have a risk factor for osteoporosis. These include:

1 patients on oral corticosteroid treatment

2   women who have had their ovaries removed before the age of 50 years
3   patients who have had a fragility fracture.

Then set up an audit to determine which patients have been appropriately screened and advised. A sample template that you could photocopy or adapt is given below. Set standards – for example, that 80% of patients with these risk factors should have a 'yes' or 'not applicable' answer to the questions.

Template for audit of prevention of osteoporosis in 'at-risk' groups

Identifier	Risk factor for osteoporosis*			Record of risk discussed in last 12 months?		Record of DEXA scan discussed in last 12 months?		Record of lifestyle advice in last 12 months?		Record of preventive medication?		
	1	2	3	Yes	No	Yes	No	Yes	No	Yes	No	N/A

* Scoring key: 1 = steroids at more than 7.5 mg daily; 2 = ovaries removed before age of 50 years; 3 = fragility fracture.
N/A = not applicable.

If your results are not good, consider setting up computer reminders to flag up risk factors during consultations. You could give patients information about the risks with repeat prescriptions and invite them to consult with a trained practice nurse, or run group information sessions. Remember to build in the intervals at which you re-audit to monitor how you are improving your results. Give feedback to all of those involved at regular intervals so that they feel rewarded for their efforts.

Exercise 16

If you are a practice manager/practice nurse/doctor, you might consider setting up guidelines for your practice and the primary care organisation (PCO) for referral for DEXA scanning, if you do not have such guidelines already. Discuss with the local provider what criteria are appropriate and put forward draft guidelines to the PCO for consultation with other practices. Once they have been set up, audit after 6 months, either in the practice, or with the provider more generally, what proportion of the referrals follow the criteria in the guidelines. Feed back the results to the practice and the PCO for discussion of whether the criteria are appropriate, or whether greater adherence to them is indicated, and plan to re-audit after any changes.

Now that you have completed one or more of the interactive reflection exercises in this chapter, transfer the information from this needs assessment to the empty templates. Use the personal development plan on pages 123–132 if you are working on your own learning plan, or the practice personal and professional development plan on pages 147–153 if you are working on a practice team learning plan. The conclusions reached at the end of each exercise will feature in the action plan. Don't forget to keep the evidence of your learning in your personal portfolio.

CHAPTER 10

Neck and shoulder pain

Neck and shoulder pain have been chosen as examples of musculo-skeletal pain to illustrate the approach you can take. You could use similar techniques to look at other common musculoskeletal conditions.

Clinical Evidence[15] has sections on plantar heel pain (including plantar fasciitis), hallux valgus (bunions) and chronic fatigue syndrome. The *Cochrane Review* (*see* list of useful websites in the Appendix) lists several systematic reviews of treatments for conditions such as acute ankle sprains and plantar heel pain. *Bandolier* (*see* list of useful websites in the Appendix) gives a review of treatments for tennis elbow, and the *Cochrane Review* is monitoring the continuing trials of treatments for this difficult-to-manage condition. The *Bandolier* review, for example, concluded that patients who had steroid injections for tennis elbow did better in the short term than those who received other treatments, but not after 6 weeks, and that pain after injection and skin atrophy might be a high price to pay for quicker relief. There were so many treatments listed that they struggled to compare them all. Thus there is no easy 'evidence-based' answer. A good account of the causes and management of knee pain in young people produced by the Arthritis and Rheumatism Council (*see* list of useful addresses and websites in the Appendix) reminds us that not all knee pain is due to cartilage injuries or osteoarthritis. Using the National Electronic Library for Health (*see* list of useful websites in the Appendix) enables you to enter a condition and search through several databases at once.

Neck pain

Neck symptoms are often diffuse and can spread into the trapezii and scapula regions. Neck pain can be divided into uncomplicated pain, whiplash, and pain with radiculopathy.[15] The causes are poorly under-stood. Most uncomplicated pain is caused by poor posture, anxiety and depression, neck strain or sport- or work-related injuries. When pain becomes chronic, the boundaries between ageing changes and causative changes to the joints are difficult to define. Just as with osteoarthritis in other areas, consider carefully whether structural changes (usually referred to as cervical spondylosis) have any relevance to the symptomatology. Cervical spondylosis is more common with increasing age of the patient, and the degree of structural change does not correlate with neck symptoms. Soft tissue injury may occur in whiplash. Rare causes of neck pain include disc prolapse and inflammatory, infective or malignant conditions with or without neurological involvement. Pain that is referred to the arm may indicate irritation or entrapment of a nerve root.

About 2% of consultations with general practitioners are for neck pain. Many more people consult chiropractors, physiotherapists or osteopaths.

Whiplash

Whiplash is a specific mechanism of injury caused by hyperextension–hyperflexion of the neck. This type of injury frequently occurs in rear-end collision and results in over-stretching and tearing of the tissues that support the head or spine. One study[49] of more than 3000 patients with whiplash injuries found that the average time to recovery was 31 days. However, recovery is likely to depend on the exact injury sustained. Another study estimated that 20–40% of patients may have persistent problems lasting longer than one year.[50] Tissues that may be injured in whiplash incidents include muscles, tendons, ligaments, intervertebral disks, blood vessels and nerves. Patient assessment includes a history, physical examination and diagnostic tests as necessary. Check whether the cervical spine has been injured if the trauma was severe.

Typical symptoms include headache, neck pain and stiffness, and back pain. Persistent pain is often complicated by other factors such as the frustration of having unresolved symptoms through no fault of their own, and long delays in resolving insurance claims. Adopt a sympathetic approach, and encourage patients to mobilise early, continue activity despite the pain, and take responsibility for their own recovery. Treat whiplash in the same way as other neck problems in order to help to reduce prolonged suffering.

Table 10.1 Systemic causes of neck pain

Inflammatory causes	Malignancy	Infection	Metabolic causes
• Ankylosing spondylitis • Rheumatoid arthritis • Polymyalgia rheumatica	• Myeloma • Metastatic disease	• Staphylococcal or other sepsis • Tuberculosis	• Osteomalacia

Systemic disease

Neck movements in systemic diseases are usually painfully limited in all directions. Possible causes are listed in Table 10.1.

Fibromyalgia

Neck pain may be part of a more generalised state of hyperalgesia, with multiple tender trigger spots together with malaise. Investigations are negative, and the symptoms may overlap with those of chronic fatigue syndrome.

Investigations

Investigations relevant to a systemic disease (*see* Chapter 2) may be necessary if more general symptoms are present. Radiography is rarely helpful. Degenerative changes are almost universal after the age of 40 years, and are usually symptomless. X-rays of the cervical spine should be reserved for presentations after acute trauma, when a bony injury may be suspected. Magnetic resonance imaging is more useful if you are considering a diagnosis of a prolapsed intervertebral disc, subluxation in rheumatoid disease, tumour, abscesses or injuries such as ruptured ligaments.

Management

One systematic review of randomised controlled trials[15] found that whiplash injuries responded to electrotherapy better than placebo, early mobilisation physiotherapy was more effective than immobilisation, and return to normal activity was better than rest. So get everyone moving!

There was insufficient evidence of the effectiveness of most physical treatments for uncomplicated neck pain.[15] Heat, cold, traction, biofeedback, spray and stretch, acupuncture and laser treatment showed no consistent improvements, but they did not show any harmful effects either. Physiotherapy and pulsed electromagnetic field therapy were found to have some beneficial effects. Mobilisation and manipulation did seem to be more effective than, for example, diazepam, non-steroidal anti-inflammatory drugs, or usual medical advice. So again, get those necks moving!

Surgical treatment was compared with conservative treatment for neck pain with neurological pain, and no difference was found at 1-year follow-up. Epidural steroid injection was only reported in case studies, so no clear conclusions could be drawn. The *ABC of Rheumatology*[26] suggests that epidural steroid injection might help to identify which patients might benefit from surgical treatment.

It is now clear that it is important to try to avoid rest and the use of cervical collars. A collar should only be used for short periods when the pain and spasm are particularly intense. Just as opinions about the role of activity in back pain have changed, evidence-based medicine provides us with the information to help to keep patients with neck pain active, too. Consider the type of work that they do when advising them about taking time off work. Prolonged sitting in one position without an opportunity to change position and mobilise the neck may be as harmful as trying to lift heavy weights above shoulder height. Occupations in which patients have control over the amount and frequency of movement may enable them to return much earlier than those in occupations where piece-work, managers or foremen drive the work routine (*see* Chapter 12 for more information on work-related considerations).

Shoulder pain

Peri-articular disorders

Clinical picture

Disorders of the rotator cuff account for most shoulder pain. In patients under 40 years of age, it usually follows over-use or injury and is due to tendinitis or rotator cuff impingement. Patients cannot lie on that shoulder at night, and complain of pain in the upper arm – demonstrating the site of the pain by clutching the lower triceps with the palm of the hand in a characteristic gesture. Examination sometimes shows the painful arc on abduction of the arm, pain on resisted movement and localised tenderness at the insertion of the rotator cuff.

Older patients may have tears of the rotator cuff, and can have severe and chronic pain.

X-rays are often not very helpful, as calcification can be seen in the supraspinatus tendon or subacromial bursa with or without shoulder pain.[26]

Pain localised at the top of the shoulder or suprascapular region suggests either a neck disorder or that the acromioclavicular joint is affected by osteoarthritis or trauma. If it is the latter, examination shows tenderness over the joint and pain on passive horizontal adduction (in contrast to rotator cuff pain). Do not forget that shoulder tip pain can also be due to gall-bladder disease, a subphrenic abscess, pulmonary embolism, or irritation of the diaphragm by residual gas following laparoscopy.

Management of rotator cuff disorders

Most cases respond to avoidance of painful movements, to non-steroidal anti-inflammatory drugs and sometimes to injections of short-acting corticosteroids and anaesthetic mixtures. Long-acting steroid injections may cause tendon rupture or soft tissue atrophy. Sleeping with a pillow under the axilla relieves some of the pain at night by supporting the weight of the arm. Tears are usually managed conservatively, but open or arthroscopic repair is sometimes performed. Physiotherapy is useful for minimising the loss of range of shoulder movement.

Acromioclavicular joint disorders

The acromioclavicular joint is easily and conveniently injected, followed by mobilisation.

Glenohumeral disorders

Clinical picture

These disorders are typically associated with loss of external rotation. Female patients complain that they cannot do up their clothing at the back, and male patients who pull off their sweaters over their heads from the back of the neck struggle to remove them for examination.

Adhesive capsulitis (frozen shoulder) presents with limitation of both active and passive movements of the shoulder, with pain at the limits of movement. Sometimes it follows a rotator cuff tear, or a systemic illness such as a myocardial infarction, lung disease or a stroke.

In patients over 50 years of age, consider polymyalgia rheumatica. Osteoarthritis of the glenohumeral joint is uncommon.

In younger patients, instability of the glenohumeral joint causes aching, and the arm is described as feeling 'dead' after throwing a ball or serving or smashing a ball or shuttlecock. Muscle-strengthening exercises are usually sufficient to improve the condition unless recurrent dislocation occurs.

Management of adhesive capsulitis

Pain relief and active movements are the mainstay of treatment, but symptoms may last for more than a year before gradual resolution. In one randomised controlled trial (RCT), distending the glenohumeral joint, in addition to intra-articular steroid injection, has been shown to increase the range of movement and reduce the severity of symptoms.[15]

Systematic reviews and RCTs have provided insufficient evidence for rating the effectiveness of most interventions in shoulder pain, largely due to the heterogenous nature of the various conditions and the lack of an accurate diagnosis.

Reflection exercises

Exercise 17

If you are a doctor/physiotherapist, you might set up a learning exercise with colleagues to improve your skills in examining the neck and shoulder joint. Ask an expert to run a practical session (e.g. a GP with a special interest, a specialist in upper limb orthopaedics or a rheumatologist). Osteopaths and physiotherapists or other doctors often have expertise that they can share with you. You could evaluate your learning by video-recording your examination of a patient or colleague before and after the learning exercise. Alternatively, if video-recording facilities are not available, ask for verbal feedback from your expert before and after the learning exercise.

Exercise 18

If you are a doctor, you might consider that having a colleague who is expert at joint and soft tissue injections in a practice (or group of practices) is a useful resource. You might wish to increase your own skills with regard to injection techniques. Check how you are doing with a suitable publication,[51] borrow a simulation model from your local postgraduate centre, attend a course, or arrange to sit in with a specialist in a clinic. Make a point of asking for feedback from others who also perform joint injections from time to time, so that you do not develop any bad habits.

Exercise 19

If you are a practice manager/ancillary staff member with responsibility for health and safety/practice or district nurse, you could produce a list of possible hazardous situations in which the neck and shoulder might be at risk, both by discussion with staff and by touring the premises with a clip-board. Look at seating by desks, reception counters, telephone points, computers and other equipment. Filing systems are a common cause of repetitive strain injury because the shelves are either too high or too low. Storing heavy items above shoulder height or in inaccessible cupboards also causes unnecessary injuries. Many nurses carry heavy equipment from room to room, or into patients' homes. Oxygen cylinders (on or off trolleys) can cause injury in the treatment room. Nurses working alone are particularly at risk from injuries caused by lifting heavy or immobile patients.

Make a list of the hazards, how commonly they cause problems, and what could be changed in order to minimise them. Present this for discussion and then implementation at a practice meeting. You might want to take this forward to the PCO as part of a strategy for an occupational health service for the PCO, or for funding for the changes to be implemented.

Now that you have completed one or more of the interactive reflection exercises in this chapter, transfer the information from this needs assessment to the empty templates. Use the personal development plan on pages 123–132 if you are working on your own learning plan, or the practice personal and professional development plan on pages 147–153 if you are working on a practice team learning plan. The conclusions reached at the end of each exercise will feature in the action plan. Don't forget to keep the evidence of your learning in your personal portfolio.

CHAPTER 11

Musculoskeletal disorders and physical disability

This chapter is based, with permission, on the booklet *One in Four of Us* produced by the Disability Partnership.[52] Musculoskeletal disorders are among the commonest causes of physical disability, particularly in older people.

Terms and models

An impairment is any loss of normal age-related structure and function of the body. Within the old, outdated medical model of disability, any consequent *disability* describes what people are unable to do as a result of an impairment, and the term *handicap* describes the social and psychological consequences of the disability. The new medical model of disability replaces the terms *disability* and *handicap* with *activities* and *participation*. It stresses the importance of environmental and other contextual influences.

Within the social model, which is preferred by many disabled people, a disability is the result of any social system that does not allow the inclusion of people with an impairment. For example, if your impairment is such that you cannot climb stairs, you are only disabled if there are places that you want to get to which offer you no alternative to access except by stairs.

Some 'people with disabilities' (a term that stresses that they are people first and disabled second) prefer to be referred to as 'disabled people', as this makes it clear that they are disabled by society's barriers. It is important to respect the terminology that people prefer, and to remember that the only expert is the person with a given disability, and that they are continually learning new ways to cope with their impairments and the barriers imposed by society.

Common causes and types of physical disability

The prevalence of physical disability increases with age. Overall, some 'one in four of us' in the UK are disabled. Only about 5–10% of young people under the age of 50 years have a disability, but the figures rise to 24% of those in the 60–69 years age bracket, 41% of those aged 70–79 years and a staggering 71% of those over 80 years of age. These data came from the Office of Population Censuses and Surveys (OPCS) survey of the 1980s,[53] but with the increasing average age of the population, the figures are probably now even higher.

Trauma and neurological disorders such as multiple sclerosis are the commonest causes in young adults, while in older people musculo-skeletal disorders, stroke, cardiovascular and respiratory disorders are the main causes of physical disability in the UK.

Some of the most frequent forms of physical impairment are listed in Box 11.1.

Box 11.1 Common forms of physical impairment[54]

Difficulty in walking (9.9%)
Hearing loss (5.9%)
Problems with personal care (5.7%)
Dexterity problems (4.0%)
Impaired vision (3.8%)
Difficulty in reaching (2.8%)
Incontinence (2.6%)

(Figures in parentheses represent the percentage of the general population in the UK.)

One person may have multiple impairments. Furthermore, one impairment may lead to another. For example, immobility may predispose to venous thrombosis or pressure sores, incontinence can cause skin problems, and drugs used to treat impairments may have disastrous side-effects.

Impairment and disability are not static – they change with time in a variety of ways, depending on the natural history of any cause (e.g. recovery from stroke), as well as individual adaptation, and the extent of people's support systems.

Support systems and carers

Support systems are critical to people with disabilities. They include family and friends, as well as money (it is expensive to be disabled) and access to services. The patient unit – family, friends and carers – should be considered as a whole.

Carers (who may be family, friends or professionals) are crucial. Their role often needs to be examined in a critical way. They sometimes want to provide help that a disabled person does not want, they may not be able to meet all of the disabled person's needs, and they may become overburdened themselves.

What is the role of the practice team?

Disability is a team issue. It involves the whole patient unit (the person with disability, and their family, friends and carers) as well as teams of professionals, including the general practitioner, practice nurse, physiotherapist, occupational therapist, pharmacist, district nurses and other supporting staff.

Some of the main roles of the practice team are outlined in Box 11.2.

Box 11.2 Some of the roles of practice team members in relation to people with disabilities

- *Listening and sharing*: being there to listen, acknowledge the problems and take the matter seriously.
- *Being the scientific expert*: being the expert on the causes of impairments and on recent medical advances, and answering the hard questions, such as 'Why me?' and 'What will happen?'.
- *Opening doors*: providing access to other professionals and organisations that can offer help.
- *Diagnosis*: identifying any complication or the cause of any change in ability or illness.
- *Symptom control*: helping to treat symptoms such as pain.
- *Secondary prevention*: predicting and helping to prevent any secondary problems, such as pressure sores or joint contractures.

Our own reactions and attitudes to people with disabilities can cause problems. The impact on us of severe disfigurement, incontinence or severe speech impairments may hamper our ability to fulfil some of the roles outlined above, and it is important that we are aware of our own problems and prejudices when we are trying to help disabled people.

Important words that may help include the following:

- *Partnership*: help for disabled people comes through partnerships between the disabled person's unit and healthcare professionals.
- *Empowerment*: our role is to help to empower those with disabilities to find the best ways of helping themselves.
- *Judgement*: beware of judgement – the disabled person is the only one who really understands their experience and problems.
- *Values*: people's values and priorities change with time, and they may be quite different to your current values, but they are no less valid.
- *Autonomy*: this should be a fundamental right of every person. Disability means a loss of some aspects of autonomy in society.
- *Listening*: this is the most important word for health professionals. Active non-judgemental listening is the core art of medicine, and is crucial for gaining an understanding of people with disabilities.
- *Shared decision making*: people with chronic conditions need to be able to make their own decisions about their management based on the expert information that is communicated to them by health professionals. Shared decision making leads to concordance.
- *Concordance*: a negotiated agreement on treatment between the patient and the healthcare professional[55] allows patients to make informed decisions with regard to the degree of risk or suffering that they themselves are willing to undertake. In contrast, 'compliance' with treatment or lifestyle changes implies that the patient follows instructions from health professionals to a greater or lesser degree.

Communicating and assessing the impact

The classical medical history involves the elicitation of symptoms with a view to making a diagnosis. In situations of chronic impairment it is more important to listen to the narrative so that you can understand the impact and share in the patient's interpretation of the meaning of their problems.[56]

There are three simple 'screening questions' that you might find helpful when trying to discover whether someone has a significant physical disability.[57] They are as follows:

1 'Do you have any difficulty in climbing stairs or steps?' (Walking difficulty is the commonest type of impairment; if you can climb steps and stairs, you can certainly walk and you can get on buses.)
2 'Do you have any difficulty in washing or dressing yourself?' (Impairments of dexterity, reaching and personal care are common, and washing and dressing are arguably the most important functional tasks to become compromised.)
3 'Do you have any difficulty with your sight or hearing?' (Hearing and visual loss are particularly common in older people.)

The use of specific self-assessment measures of disability or quality of life may occasionally be helpful, but listening to the patient's narrative and getting to grips with what really matters to them is much more valuable.

Consider the following examples.

Assessing a patient with rheumatoid arthritis

The patient's narrative

Well, I was managing OK, I suppose, until Christmas. Christmas is always difficult. I feel I ought to be making it special for the children, but this year the pain was so bad that I just could not cope with the cooking and decorating. John [husband] was supportive, but I felt it was flat, and the kids got upset and argued a lot. I felt very depressed afterwards. I thought I had let everyone down. Then my wrists started hurting more and I dropped one of John's special glasses and broke it. Now I am really worried. It might all be slipping away from me. What will John do? Will he stay with us? I feel awful.

I am also worried about Sarah [daughter]. Will I give the arthritis to her? What is happening to us? I won't let Sarah play near the river because I am convinced that my arthritis is due to the wet I was exposed to when I was her age. But she does not understand. What is happening to us?

The medical notes

46-year-old with long-standing RA. Married with two children. Routine review shows low joint score (18) with active right wrist, but no new systemic features or signs. ESR is 46. HAQ (a self-assessment measure of disability) low at only 1.4. Advised to increase dose of methotrexate to 15 mg weekly, and to continue as before. To be seen in another 4 months when we might consider injecting the right wrist.

The new patient

A man in his late thirties who has just joined the practice comes to see you for the first time. He has cerebral palsy. You have great difficulty in understanding him and are distracted by his athetoid movements. You finally realise that he wants advice about the use of prophylactic aspirin for heart disease. You provide the advice.

Afterwards you say to your practice nurse 'Poor chap, so disabled'. Your nurse replies 'Oh, didn't you know? That's the new University Professor of Anthropology, and what's more he is the new coach for their sailing team'.

The old patient

An old friend of the practice recently had a mild stroke. After discharge from hospital he comes to visit you. You examine him carefully and cannot find much wrong. After he has gone, you say to a colleague 'Old Fred seems to have had a lucky escape from his stroke – hardly any residual disability at all'.

Fred leaves your surgery in a very despondent state of mind. He finds his way to the bank. Since his stroke he has lost his wife (who had an affair with one of the neighbours) and he has run up a large bank overdraft as a result of lost work and the expense of being disabled.

The doctors failed to assess accurately or understand the disabilities of any of these three patients, although in each case, had they listened to the narrative properly, they would not have made these mistaken assumptions.

Difficulties in the assessment of people with disabilities can also arise when we forget that they are just as likely to contract a disease as anyone else. It is all too easy to forget to make sure that someone who is confined to their home gets their cervical smear, or to check the blood pressure of that angry chap in the wheelchair who is always ranting on about the way in which the medical profession has failed him.

Hidden disabilities

Disabilities are often hidden, and some people are distressed by the fact that their peer group or others think that they are perfectly healthy.

Here are some examples.

> A 57-year-old man with ischaemic heart disease looks fit but cannot get upstairs because of shortness of breath. A passer-by asks him to help a disabled person get their wheelchair up some steps. He cannot do this. The passer-by sneers and says 'Huh, fit able-bodied chap like you not willing to help a disabled person – what is the country coming to?'.

> A 36-year-old man with diabetes is ostracised at work because he won't go out to the pub for lunch on Fridays with his workmates or join in the regular beer and curry evenings because he cannot take this risk.

> A 44-year-old Asian woman with epilepsy is having trouble getting a job in her chosen career as a sales representative because she cannot drive.

> A 36-year-old man who is HIV-positive is so frightened of passing the condition on to others that he avoids many 'normal' situations for fear of cutting himself and blood being spilt.

Each of these people has a significant 'hidden disability'.

Summary

Dealing with people with disabilities is both challenging and exciting. Some of the key points within this chapter are summarised in Box 11.3.

Box 11.3 Points to remember about disability

- Very few diseases can be cured. Most people have to live with the consequences of disease.
- Disability is common. About one in four people in the UK is either disabled or caring for someone with a disability.
- Disability should be integral to education and training in medicine.
- Disability should be central to the provision of services and care.
- Good communication (especially listening) is the key to understanding and assessing disability.
- Disability has as much to do with the environment as with impairment.
- Think about the carer as well as the disabled person.
- The individual with disability is the only real expert on their disability.
- Disabled people are individuals who are just as likely to get other diseases as anyone else.
- Partnerships facilitate empowerment and autonomy.
- Avoid making assumptions.
- Try to accept other people's values and beliefs when providing care.

Reflection exercises

Exercise 20

Any member of the practice team could find out more about what it feels like to be a person with a physical disability visiting your practice. Ask one or two of your most disabled patients to walk with you around the surgery premises and to point out the hazards and difficulties for them. Look at access to the surgery itself and to the toilets, public telephone and reception desk. Are all of the public rooms accessible? Is the disabled person's choice of GP or nurse limited by where the consulting-rooms are sited (e.g. on the first floor without a lift)? What aids and equipment are there for helping immobile people up on to an examination couch? Do you have any equipment for visually impaired patients or those who are hard of hearing? Are children's toys stored away from gangways so that disabled people have an unobstructed path around the waiting-room?

Make a list of the obstructions and hazards, and draw up an action plan to rectify these. Do you need to learn more about how to anticipate and accommodate the needs of people with physical disabilities?

Exercise 21

As a GP or practice nurse, you could review what you know about grading the extent of disability of a person with a mobility, visual, auditory or functional disability. We used three screening questions in this chapter, but you should have a look at other measures of function,[58] such as the Barthel index and the Aids to Daily Living functional scale.

If you are not familiar with these, you could ask your local community physiotherapist or occupational therapist to run an informal teaching session in the practice. Alternatively, sit in with your local rheumatologist for a couple of sessions and pick his or her brains, or read up about disability in the library. Then you could reach a consensus with all of the clinical staff in the practice about how you will rate disability in future. Include GPs, practice nurses and district nurses in the decision making.

Now that you have completed one or more of the interactive reflection exercises in this chapter, transfer the information from this needs assessment to the empty templates. Use the personal development plan on pages 123–132 if you are working on your own learning plan, or the practice personal and professional development plan on pages 147–153 if you are working on a practice team learning plan. The conclusions reached at the end of each exercise will feature in the action plan. Don't forget to keep the evidence of your learning in your personal portfolio.

CHAPTER 12

Disability and employment

This chapter is based on extracts from *Occupational Health Matters in General Practice.*[21]*

Rehabilitation, resettlement and retirement

Rehabilitation in occupational health terms simply means getting the worker back to work in a job that is appropriate to their medical condition – by temporary or permanent redeployment, or by specific redesign of the job. Communication between the employer or occupational health service and the GP is of great help. The GP has knowledge of specific medical factors that may limit a patient temporarily or permanently, and may also have background information on hospital investigations, treatment and rehabilitation after illness or injury.

Ill-health retirement may be necessary if the worker is permanently unable to do the job for which they were contracted and no suitable alternative can be found. Discussion between the occupational physician and the individual's GP is important before considering ill-health retirement. Careful thought must be given to the physical and psychological consequences, including the possible financial difficulties. Both the GP and the occupational physician need to have a working knowledge of the sickness and disability benefits available so that they can help the patient to make an appropriate claim.

Permanent disability need not be a bar to future employment (*see* Box 12.1).

* Dr Philip Sawney, Medical Policy Manager at the Department of Social Security, contributed to the original text as well as the authors of the book.

Box 12.1

- Retirement from their regular occupation on the grounds of ill health or disability does not mean that the person cannot continue to work.
- A range of employment-related services available to GPs and their patients are aimed at maximising work potential and giving people an opportunity to continue to make a positive contribution whenever possible (details are provided in the *IB204 Guide* issued by the Department of Social Security[59] to all GPs).
- State sickness benefits such as the Incapacity Benefit can often be a far less attractive option than more active intervention on the part of the GP, the patient and the occupational health services.

Specific problems

Workers with certain conditions need special consideration with regard to their fitness to work. The cases described in Boxes 12.2 and 12.3 illustrate how such conditions might be approached.

Box 12.2

A 38-year-old man with a rotator cuff injury to his right shoulder asks your advice as to whether he should enter training as an ambulance driver. (He has recovered full movements but cannot continue in his previous employment, as it involves very heavy lifting that caused his injury.) He tells you that the job specification states that he would be working with a partner so will not have to do any lifting on his own. He has done voluntary work in the St John's Ambulance Service for many years and sees this as a suitable alternative employment for which he already has some skills. What clinical and occupational issues would you take into account when advising him?

There are wider implications than the simple clinical issues here. This man may now feel that he is completely fit for ordinary duties, but he may be called upon to assist at accidents where he might have to lift someone on his own, or to lift heavy and immobile patients in the home in awkward situations where two people cannot reach. He may not feel able to carry out an activity that is likely to cause his shoulder further damage. He has to consider what a patient's reaction would be if he was called to an emergency and then could not manage because of his previous injury. He may meet prejudice or anxiety from managers and colleagues if he is not reliably able to carry out his duties.

This is where the GP's knowledge of the patient and their medical problems can be used in conjunction with the occupational health department, covering all the points listed above, and giving the patient and their prospective trainers/employers advice on their suitability for a particular job. It may be possible to utilise this man's skills within the ambulance service, but perhaps not in the front-line, where his disability could hinder his effectiveness.

Box 12.3

A 63-year-old woman has developed polymyalgia rheumatica and is now very much better on high-dose steroids. She wishes to return to work but seeks your advice. She works in a hospital microbiological laboratory processing the identification of types of infection in human samples, and is concerned about her greater susceptibility to infection. She is also worried that she might be at risk of being compulsorily retired or sacked because of her health risks, and is concerned about the effect that this would have on her pension which she wishes to take at the age of 65 years.

It is easiest to relieve this woman's anxieties about her second worry. Unless she is unable to do her work through her ill health, then her employers do not have grounds to dismiss her. (Exceptions to this would be if her contract of employment stipulates an age of retirement before 65 years, or if she has a fixed-term contract of employment that expires before then – and neither of these would be affected by her health status.) If she is unable to do her work due to ill health (e.g. if she had a relapse or developed a complication), retirement due to ill health usually includes an upgrading of the pension. She would need to consult her pension officer at work to establish the exact position for her circumstances, but she would probably find that at her age she would receive the same pension as she would expect to receive at retirement age.

There should be strict rules in force in the laboratory about the handling of infectious samples. The Health and Safety Executive regulations should be available in the workplace. The occupational health department of the hospital should be aware of any special problems, and the GP and occupational health officer should be able to consult together over any extra health risk to which this patient might be exposed. Modifications to her working environment could be made if necessary. In any case, the occupational health department will want to be fully informed about her absence from work and any requirements necessary when she returns to work. The patient should arrange to see them and her GP should discuss with her what information she wants them to receive from her medical records to enable him or her to prepare a helpful report.

Some jobs have particularly strict health requirements. These include commercial driving and flying, offshore work or seafaring and professional diving. Good advice to the patient and prospective employer is essential in order to avoid problems.[60] A 57-year-old man with osteoarthritis of the hips and knees may be able to manage to drive his family to see the in-laws, but may not be able to manage a journey across Europe sleeping in the cab of his car transporter at night.

Beneficial effects of work

It is too easy to assume that all effects of work on health must be negative. In fact, having a job has major psychosocial benefits, with secondary beneficial effects on physical health. Unemployment is associated with psychological morbidity (low self-esteem, chronic depression), and employment provides the financial basis for good nutrition and hygiene. Physically demanding jobs help to maintain muscular fitness and stamina, together with general cardiorespiratory fitness.

In general, an employer's health and safety policy and the management systems that are in place to implement and audit compliance with the policy contribute to the health and safety of the workforce. In addition, an employer may introduce the following:

- no-smoking policies at work
- subsidised canteen food and 'healthy eating' options
- on-site (or subsidised) exercise or gym facilities, with inducements and encouragement for participants
- general health screening (blood pressure, cholesterol, etc.)
- employment policies which encourage individuals to control their work and reduce stress.

Occupational health services have a direct role in health promotion. They may initiate or support general health promotion (e.g. diet, smoking, exercise) and may be involved in specific projects that are related more to the hazards which are encountered at work. Education of the workforce in matters of health, hygiene and accident prevention is important.

The involvement of occupational health services in general health screening is more controversial. Is it appropriate for occupational health services to undertake screening for risk factors (e.g. smoking habits, blood pressure, cholesterol, diabetes, etc.)? Is it appropriate for them to undertake cancer screening such as cervical cytology or prostate-specific antigen testing in the workplace?

If an occupational health doctor or nurse finds a raised ESR on 'health screening', then it is vital to counsel the individual and communicate the results to the GP, but it is still the GP who has responsibility for following up an abnormal result and for prescribing. GPs may have concerns about occupational health services undertaking these tasks unless they are satisfied with regard to the quality of the service, the confidentiality of the results, and the communication and follow-up of abnormalities.

Demands of work – disability, chronic ill health, rehabilitation and resettlement and ill-health retirement

Disability and chronic ill health

The Disability Discrimination Act (1995) makes it illegal for employers of 15 or more staff to discriminate against people with disabilities when selecting, training or promoting employees.[61,62] It requires employers to make reasonable changes to the workplace to accommodate people with disabilities and to help them to work. In this context, disability is defined as any physical, sensory or mental condition that makes it difficult for the person to carry out normal day-to-day activities and that is likely to last for more than 12 months. It will also include conditions that currently have only a slight effect on day-to-day activities, but the effects of which are expected to become more substantial (e.g. rheumatoid arthritis).

Box 12.4

Contrast these two situations and consider whether ill-health retirement might be recommended for:

(i) a 28-year-old secretary with neck pain following a whiplash injury

(ii) a 57-year-old postman with osteoarthritis of both hips.

In case (i) it should be possible to modify the secretary's job to avoid exacerbating her neck problems, but in case (ii) the postman is likely to be permanently unfit to continue work as a postman, unless redeployment into a sedentary job is possible.

Ill-health retirement may be necessary in some situations, where illness or injury are so significant that redeployment and resettlement are impossible. An employer is entitled to dismiss an employee on the grounds of ill health, and an employee who is a member of a pension scheme is entitled to ask for early retirement with full pension benefits. Pension fund trustees usually require some kind of medical certification that the person is 'unfit', but the exact rules vary from one scheme to another.

Some pension schemes simply require the employee to be unfit to do their usual job or any comparable job. Some pension schemes are more prescriptive, and may require certification of permanent incapacity to do any type of work.

The Personal Capability Assessment (PCA) introduced in April 2000 focuses on residual capabilities, rather than just 'incapacity'. The postman may well be able to undertake another form of work that is less physically exacting. Medical advice to inform benefit decision making is provided by a doctor 'approved' by the Secretary of State for Social Security, and not the GP or the occupational physician.

In assessing whether the changes they could make to the workplace or to the way in which the work is done are 'reasonable', the employer is allowed to take into account how much the changes would cost and how much they would help. The Act does not apply to operational staff employed in the armed forces, the police, the prison services, the fire services, or to anyone employed on board ships, hovercraft or aeroplanes.

Employment legislation prior to the Disability Discrimination Act (DDA) required employers of more than 20 people to have a quota of 3% disabled – a quota that was frequently not filled.

Many patients with disabilities did not register as disabled under the 'old' system. In terms of job prospects, there are both advantages and disadvantages to an individual if they admit that they have a 'disability'.

Up to the introduction of the Disability Discrimination legislation, there were two occupations reserved for individuals who were registered disabled, namely car park attendant and electric lift attendant, although positive discrimination for other jobs by enlightened employers (or employers wishing to fulfil their quota of 3% disabled under the old scheme) was possible.

However, negative discrimination by many employers who still do not attempt to accommodate disabled employees leads many people with 'disabilities' to try to make light of them or even deny them altogether.

The DDA legislation is aimed at giving disabled people a fair chance of employment in all jobs, and should encourage applicants to acknowledge their physical or psychological limitations in the knowledge that they will be treated fairly.

Employment *helps* a disabled person, or one with a chronic illness, through the general benefits of work, together with improved morale and self-image for those who are able to be productive in paid employment despite having a disability.

Box 12.5

Compare the following two situations and consider whether ill health retirement might be recommended for:

(i) a 52-year-old chemical process worker with systemic lupus erythematosus, on maximum doses of inhaled medication, and whose chest symptoms are exacerbated by exposure to chemical fumes

(ii) a 45-year-old forestry worker who has had a hip replacement for early-onset osteoarthritis.

Redeployment and retraining should be possible in both cases, even if the employees are unable to return to their old jobs or old employers, so the pension fund rules may preclude them from drawing their pension.

If you are asked for your opinion on ill-health retirement, either directly by Pension Fund Trustees or indirectly by an occupational physician, it might be necessary to ask about the rules in detail before commenting on your patient's long-term prognosis. If the rules are very strict, the patient may find him- or herself without a job, and without an ill-health pension.

Rehabilitation and resettlement

An appreciation of the role of occupational health services and other agencies in resettlement and rehabilitation is very important for the general practitioner and practice nurse. It is not uncommon for a patient with a chronic medical problem to believe that they cannot or should not return to work, and for their GP to issue sick notes without considering the options for rehabilitation and resettlement. For a patient who is claiming a state incapacity benefit, the GP will not have to issue further statements following the medical assessment by the DSS Benefits Agency. This will usually be at around six months into a spell of incapacity, but is increasingly being applied earlier.

A GP has access to a number of agencies to help to get their patients back to work after illness or injury, including the employer's occupational health service (where there is one). Variables such as hours of work, physical and psychological demands and workstation design are critical. Advice on these matters (and the pace at which someone should be brought back up to 'full speed' at work) can be given to management by an occupational health service with additional advice from other services.

Advice from occupational therapy departments may be helpful when considering physical adaptations to workstations or aids to mobility.

Every Job Centre has a Disability Employment Adviser (DEA) who can give advice on all aspects of employment, and who has contacts with employers and training agencies. The service of the DEA is open to those who are in employment as well as to the unemployed. For those under 18 years of age, the local Careers Service deals with questions of employment and disability, and this may be vital advice for a patient with juvenile arthritis who needs to plan what type of employment is going to be possible.

Box 12.6

A 42-year-old hospital porter suffered an episode of neck pain with referred pain in the arm. The GP advised a short period of rest, followed by mobilisation and physiotherapy. After a month the porter's neck pain had not entirely settled, and he went back to his GP for another sick note (Med 3). The GP might liaise with the occupational health service or DEA as an alternative to issuing another sickness certificate.

Occupational physicians know that the pressures on a GP's time are great. It is neither easy nor always feasible to negotiate resettlement and temporary (or permanent) redeployment for your patients within the time that you have available. Issuing a further sickness certificate (Med 3) to a patient who says 'I don't think I'm ready to go back to that job, doc' is a responsible response. Naturally, the patient's *attitude* to returning to work is vital, but if there is an occupational health service to assist with assessment of the workplace and work demands in relation to residual disability – and/or referral to the Regional Disability Service is feasible – then getting the patient back to work quickly becomes a real possibility.

In general, a patient may not be well served in the longer term by medical advice to refrain from work, if more appropriate clinical management would allow them to stay in work or to return to work as quickly as is reasonably practicable. In this case, when providing advice to a patient about their fitness for work, the GP may wish to consider the following factors:

- the nature of the patient's medical condition and how long the condition is expected to last
- the functional limitations which result from the patient's condition, particularly in relation to the types of tasks they actually perform at work
- any reasonable adjustments which might enable the patient to continue working
- any appropriate clinical guidelines (*see* appropriate chapters in this book)

- clinical management of the condition which is in the patient's best interest with regard to work fitness
- how to manage the patient's expectations in relation to their ability to continue working.

Employers, occupational health services and the DEA can refer individuals to the Regional Disability Service for further advice. These specialist teams can arrange assessment of physical or psychological problems. For example, one common reason for referral is chronic pain. They assess the client's aptitude for – and attitude towards – certain types of work, and counselling by occupational psychologists can aid appropriate redeployment at work. Further training and job rehearsal can be arranged. The Regional Disability Service (like occupational therapists) has access to a wide range of aids that may facilitate return to work.

Box 12.7

The types of aids and modifications that might help a secretary with severe rheumatoid arthritis to stay at work include the following:

- modifications to visual display units (VDUs) and workstations
- special keyboards
- modified pointing devices
- voice-activated word-processing systems
- special seating or adaptations for wheelchairs
- aids to assist the handling of paper and files
- help with transport to work
- adaptations to cars.

Other aids are available, including large screens, magnifying equipment, etc. Communication aids for the deaf and deafened, and help with transport (adaptations to a car or help with costs of taxi fares for employees who cannot use public transport) can be arranged.

Under the Access to Work scheme, costs of adaptations to the work environment, including the introduction of new equipment, can be covered (or partially covered) by grants from the Regional Disability Service or DEA. For example, for employees with poor visual acuity, magnifying screens or large screens can be provided for VDU work at a reduced cost to the employer.

Fitness for work and health screening

Pre-employment assessment

When a doctor is asked to assess fitness for a particular job at pre-employment stage, either by medical examination or by health questionnaire, the primary responsibility is to the employer. Any information given to the employer is only in terms of 'fitness to work'.

Occasionally an occupational health service will ask the individual's GP for a report at the pre-employment stage, justified by anxiety over potentially concealed but significant illness. Whenever the occupational physician is asking for a report in these circumstances, they should be clear about why the information is necessary, and should seek the person's *informed* written consent, rather than relying on a brief consent form that a job applicant is hardly likely to refuse to sign.

GPs are likely to receive such requests for information from time to time, and their reports will be used to help the occupational health service to advise management, bearing in mind the provisions of the Disability Discrimination Act. Any report therefore needs to be based on a real understanding of the job concerned. The onus is on the potential employer who is requesting the report to make the GP aware of any specific requirements of the job that may have a bearing on their patient's fitness.

Management referral after absence attributed to sickness

The occupational physician's responsibility is primarily to the employee when assessing someone with a poor sickness absence record. Care must be taken to ensure that the employee understands the doctor's role, and that management are not using the doctor to put pressure on an employee. The control of absence attributed to sickness is a legitimate interest of occupational health departments, but is a *management* responsibility. In the case of an employee referred under specific disciplinary procedures (e.g. drug and alcohol abuse policies), the doctor must make it clear to the individual precisely what the purpose of the referral is and what management expects.

Ill-health retirement

Occupational physicians are alert to the possibility of being used to shed unwanted labour via the ill-health retirement route rather than via redundancy. They should understand the provisions of the company's pension scheme and should be familiar with the state benefits that may apply. Occupational health doctors should always give impartial advice and not be swayed either by an employer's pressure or by the employee's wishes. They should also be prepared to collect supporting evidence of being permanently unfit to work (with the worker's consent) from GPs and hospital specialists. This is one area where communication with the GP is vital in order to ensure co-operation and support. Moreover, it is essential that the occupational physician and GP remember that a person who is unfit for a particular job is not necessarily unfit for all work (as discussed before). It is important that patients are not wrongly advised to think that if the GP is prepared to issue sickness absence certificates they will continue to receive a state incapacity benefit.

Apart from the GP being asked whether to support ill-health retirement for one of their patients (and this usually implies continuing to issue sickness absence certificates), he or she may very occasionally be asked in confidence about the prognosis of life-threatening illness. Many pension schemes have a clause that allows members to waive their pension in favour of a large lump sum on retirement. This option is not usually worthwhile, but if someone knows that they have only a few months to live, signing a 'commutation of pension' may give their family a very substantial lump sum. Clearly this may be a delicate matter because the patient may not know (or may not want to know) their prognosis. If you feel that they should not be told that they have a very poor prognosis, even if this means a loss of pension, this information is very important to the occupational physician and the pension fund trustees, who will want to give the patient the best possible financial outcome.

Disability Discrimination Act 1995 (DDA)

The section of this Act which relates to employment and places obligations on employers only applies to businesses which employ 15 or more employees. As such it may only apply to larger general practices. However, the principles of the Act embody good employment practice and should therefore be followed irrespective of practice size. The Act makes it unlawful for employers to discriminate against current or prospective employees with disabilities on account of their disability.

This applies in the following areas:

- recruitment (i.e. at pre-employment assessment)
- promotion
- training and development
- dismissal.

The Disability Discrimination Act[62] covers people with a past disability as well as a present one, and that disability is defined as 'a physical or mental impairment which has a substantial and long-term adverse effect on a person's ability to carry out normal day-to-day activities'.

Employers must also make reasonable changes to premises, work practices and employment arrangements (e.g. hours of work and work breaks) in order to accommodate a disabled employee.

Long-term effects include those that have lasted or are likely to last for 12 months or more, whether continuously or by periodic recurrence. Normal day-to-day activities cover the following broad categories:

- mobility
- manual dexterity
- physical co-ordination
- continence
- ability to lift, carry or move ordinary objects
- speech, hearing or eyesight
- memory, or ability to concentrate, learn or understand
- being able to recognise physical dangers.

Reflection exercises

Exercise 22

As a receptionist, you might identify a learning need to be better informed about the requirement for sickness certification. Get together with your work colleagues and record the questions that patients ask you. Find out from your manager how to collect the information that you and your colleagues need in order to improve the accuracy of your advice, or where patients themselves can access the advice that they need. Your local Citizens' Advice Bureau and Department of Social Security Office may also be able to advise you about suitable information sources, such as leaflets.

Exercise 23

As a manager, you might identify a learning need to be better informed about the Disability Discrimination Act or Health and Safety regulations. Your primary care organisation or the practice managers' association may be able to help with suitable courses or information.

Exercise 24

As a health professional, you might identify a learning need to be better informed about the role of occupational health services. Consider meeting for discussion with, or shadowing for a couple of days (selected for variations in the work), a colleague who works in occupational health.

Now that you have completed one or more of the interactive reflection exercises in this chapter, transfer the information from this needs assessment to the empty templates. Use the personal development plan on pages 123–132 if you are working on your own learning plan, or the practice personal and professional development plan on pages 147–153 if you are working on a practice team learning plan. The conclusions reached at the end of each exercise will feature in the action plan. Don't forget to keep the evidence of your learning in your personal portfolio.

CHAPTER 13

Draw up and apply your personal development plan

You may be interested in making the improvement of your prevention and management of musculoskeletal disorders a focus of your personal development plan (PDP). A PDP on the prevention and management of musculoskeletal disorders could supplement a practice personal and professional development plan on musculoskeletal disorders (see Chapter 14). Therefore we have included a worked example of a personal development plan focused on the prevention and management of musculoskeletal disorders on pages 133–144.

The example given is very comprehensive, and you may not want to include so much in your own personal development plan. You might include different topics and educational activities, because your needs and circumstances are different to those of the example practitioner described here. You might want to spend half of your available time on this topic and the rest on other priority subjects, such as those in National Service Frameworks, or topics from your local or district health improvement plan.

You need to involve your colleagues and workplace team in anything that you propose to include in your own personal development plan. Some suggestions are included in the example. You should also discuss it with your education and clinical governance leads in your own workplace. They will be able to help you to focus down on to achievable aims and objectives, and point out any gaps you might not have thought about as well. Your personal development plan also needs to feed into the practice or workplace development plans, so consult as widely as possible before you start. Keep it simple, so that after a year you will be able to measure some progress. Then you can build on that, or change focus for a while, in subsequent years.

Transfer the information about your learning needs from any of the reflection exercises at the end of the chapters that are relevant to you and that you have completed to the empty template of the personal development plan that follows on pages 123–132. The reflection exercises that you choose to select will depend on the focus of your PDP – as in the worked example here or other facets of musculoskeletal disorders.

The conclusions you have reached at the end of each exercise will feature in the action plan of your personal development plan. Some more ideas about the preliminary information you should be gathering for your personal development plan are given in the boxes of the template. The template, and other examples of development plans, are available on the Primary Care Online website (*see* list of useful websites in the Appendix).

Template for your personal development plan

Photocopy the following pages and complete one chart per topic.

What topic have you chosen?

Who chose it?

Justify why the topic is a priority:

(i) *A personal or professional priority?*

(ii) *A practice priority?*

(iii) *A district priority?*

(iv) *A national priority?*

Who will be included in your personal development plan?
(Anyone other than you? GPs, employed staff, attached staff, others from outside the practice, patients?)

What baseline information will you collect and how?

How will you identify your learning needs?
(How will you obtain this information and who will do it? Self-completion check-lists, discussion, appraisal, audit, patient feedback?)

What are the learning needs of your practice or workplace and how do they match your needs?

Is there any patient or public input to your personal development plan?

Aims of your personal development plan arising from the preliminary data-gathering exercise:

How might you integrate the 14 components of clinical governance into your personal development plan, focusing on the topic of . . . . ?

Establishing a learning culture:

Managing resources and services:

Establishing a research and development culture:

Reliable and accurate data:

Evidence-based practice and policy:

Confidentiality:

Health gain:

Coherent team:

Audit and evaluation:

Meaningful involvement of patients and the public:

Health promotion:

Risk management:

Accountability and performance:

Core requirements:

Action plan (include the objectives above, timetabled action and expected outcomes)

How does your personal development plan tie in with your other strategic plans? (e.g. the practice's business or development plan, the local health improvement programme, or the primary care investment plan)

What additional resources will you require to execute your plan and from where do you hope to obtain them?
(Will you have to pay any course fees? Will you be able to organise any protected time for learning in working hours?)

How will you evaluate your personal development plan?

How will you know when you have achieved your objectives?
(How will you measure success?)

How will you disseminate the learning from your plan to the rest of your team and patients? How will you sustain your new-found knowledge or skills?

How will you handle new learning requirements as they crop up?

Check whether the topic you have chosen is a priority and the way in which you plan to learn about it is appropriate.

Photocopy this pro forma for future use.

Your topic:

How have you identified your learning need(s)?

(*a*) PCO requirement	☐	(*e*) Appraisal need	☐
(*b*) Practice business plan	☐	(*f*) New to post	☐
(*c*) Legal mandatory requirement	☐	(*g*) Individual decision	☐
(*d*) Job requirement	☐	(*h*) Patient feedback	☐
		(*i*) Other	☐

. . . .

Have you discussed or planned your learning needs with anyone else?

Yes ☐   No ☐   If yes, who?

. . . .

What are your learning need(s) and/or objective(s) in terms of the following?

Knowledge. What new information do you hope to gain to help you to do this?

. . . .

Skills. What should you be able to do differently as a result of undertaking this learning in your development plan?

. . . .

Behaviour/professional practice. How will this impact on the way in which you then do things?

. . . .

Details and date of desired development activity:

. . . .

Details of any previous training and/or experience you have in this area/dates:

. . . .

What is your current performance in this area compared with the requirements of your job?

Need significant ☐   Need some ☐
development in this area   development in this area

Satisfactory in this area ☐   Do well in this area ☐

What is the level of job relevance that this area has to your role and responsibilities?

Has no relevance to job ☐   Has some relevance ☐

Relevant to job ☐   Very relevant ☐

Essential to job ☐

Describe how the proposed education/training is relevant to your job:

. . . .

Do you need additional support in identifying a suitable development activity?

Yes ☐   No ☐

What do you need?

. . . .

Describe the differences or improvements for you, your practice, PCO and/or NHS trust as a result of undertaking this activity:

. . . .

Assess the priority of your proposed educational/training activity:

Urgent ☐   High ☐   Medium ☐   Low ☐

Describe how the proposed activity will meet your learning needs rather than any other type of course or training on the topic:

. . . .

If you had a free choice, would you want to learn this? Yes/No

If **No**, why not? (please circle all that apply):

Waste of time
I have already done it
It is not relevant to my work or career goals
Other

If **Yes**, what reasons are most important to you? (put them in rank order):

To improve my performance
To increase my knowledge
To get promotion
I am just interested in it
To be better than my colleagues
To do a more interesting job
To enable me to be more confident
Because it will help me

Record of your learning

Write in the topic, date and time spent for each type of learning

	Activity 1	Activity 2	Activity 3	Activity 4
In-house formal learning				
External courses				
Informal and personal				
Qualifications and/or experience gained				

Worked example of a personal development plan: the prevention and management of musculoskeletal disorders

Who chose the topic?

It might be your own choice or that of someone in the practice team or PCO team who thinks that you should have additional skills in the prevention and management of musculoskeletal disorders.

Why is the topic a priority?:

(i) *A personal or professional priority*? You may have chosen the prevention and management of musculoskeletal disorders, seeing a need for it yourself or as an inevitable development in your work. You may have agreed as part of your work development, or as a requirement of a change in work duties or responsibilities. You may have volunteered after development in the prevention and management of musculoskeletal disorders was identified as a practice or PCO need.

(ii) *A practice priority*? The practice may have a need for an in-house expert to provide best practice and reduce costs. Perhaps the practice has identified that members of staff have been away from work, or unable to do their work as usual because of musculoskeletal symptoms. You may have received a complaint or had a patient of yours subject to a critical incident analysis. Patient need or a different skill mix in the practice may have increased the need for expertise in the prevention and management of musculoskeletal disorders.

(iii) *A district priority*? The PCO may need a local expert to provide guidelines and services. They may be concerned about high referral rates to secondary care or high prescribing levels in the area.

(iv) *A national priority*? The reduction of time off work and the prevention of disability are important national priorities.

Who will be included in your personal development plan?

You might like to find others who want to develop their skills. Working together or establishing a cascade of learning from each other makes learning more cost-effective and you can set consistent standards of care. Learning skills and then passing them on makes for more effective learning for you, too.

Everyone needs to have the opportunity – reception staff, the practice manager, secretaries, *all* of the health professionals and anyone who uses your premises might benefit from the prevention and management of musculoskeletal disorders. Disseminating basic information may reduce the workload of health professionals. Remember confidentiality and security issues.

You may want to consider training as a PCO activity to ensure consistency, exchange skills and reduce costs. Bringing in outside experts then becomes more cost-effective and can be tailor-made for the particular needs of the learning group.

Who will collect the baseline information and how?

You could ask the practice manager or secretary, or the clinical tutor at the PCO, the rheumatology or Accident and Emergency departments, the physiotherapy and occupational health and therapy departments, etc., for details of the training that is available. If you are already connected to the Internet, you can search for other, more distant information yourself.

You need to know what is being done at present, so set up an audit of your current management. Find out the number of incidents of work-related injury in your practice, and in other practices in your PCO. The occupational health doctor at an industrial site in your practice area may be prepared to share their records with you, provided that they are anonymised. Find out what guidelines for the management of musculo-skeletal disorders are already available.

Find out what is in the pipeline for the immediate and long-term future development of the prevention and management of musculo-skeletal disorders in your area.

How will you identify your learning needs?

You could keep a record of patient queries or situations where you lacked enough knowledge to deal with them skilfully. Among other methods you might want to perform a SWOT analysis for yourself and with your practice team, as follows.

- *Strengths*: Enthusiasm. An interest in sports and sports medicine. Willingness to go on learning. Communication skills and inter-professional relationships to enable inter-disciplinary working. Organisational skills, teaching skills, and research skills to provide a resource for the management of preventive and treatment mea-sures. A practice with sufficient spare capacity for quality improve-ments and to provide a resource for the PCO.
- *Opportunities*: A contact in health and leisure provision for the locality. An individual with skills in the prevention and manage-ment of musculoskeletal disorders, who is enthusiastic about passing

on his or her newly acquired knowledge. Expertise in evaluating interventions on which you can build for professional proficiency. A decision to gain expertise in prevention.

- *Weaknesses and threats*: Deficiencies in equipment, time for performing interventions, and deficiencies in the availability of training. Too many guidelines and increasing numbers of National Service Framework requirements for the practice team to meet. Other commitments, antagonism or lack of support from others.

You might include a survey of the expertise available in your PCO and elsewhere and list the present competencies of other staff. What skills and services are accessible inside and outside your own workplace?

What are the learning needs of the practice and how do they match your needs?

The reflection exercises should have already given you some information. Consider inviting people to express their concerns and opinions at a practice team meeting, or ask another member of staff to organise this. The practice manager could ask people to complete a check-list of their own needs and wishes with regard to the prevention and management of musculoskeletal disorders, and what they would like from others.

One staff member might wish to specialise and become an expert in the prevention and management of musculoskeletal disorders. Does that fit with the requirements of the practice (or PCO)? Would it be more cost-effective to obtain that expertise from another practice?

A GP might wish to become a clinical assistant in secondary care or an intermediate care provider for the PCO. What implications does this have for the practice in terms of cover for clinical sessions?

A practice nurse might wish to gain expertise in counselling people with long-term musculoskeletal problems, or in the prevention of injuries in older people. What implications does this have for her other workload?

You might find that your local physiotherapist wishes to take over more of the management of acute and chronic musculoskeletal disorders. Does this have implications for your budget and waiting-list for other conditions?

You might wish to employ an osteopath or chiropractor, or provide space for one to work independently at your practice. What does this mean for your patients? Can you recommend patients to attend? Who will pay for the service? Will it be independent or managed by the practice? Will you need to make alterations to the layout of your premises or to the equipment used? How will these be financed? Do you know what their qualifications are and if they are accredited by a professional body?

You might like the PCO to purchase (or arrange to use independently) sessions at a local gym or health club for prevention training and rehabilitation.

You may want to work with a local residential or nursing home to prevent and treat musculoskeletal disorders among their staff or residents. Will this require renegotiation of your contract of services with the home?

Is there any patient or public input to your plan?

You may well have some local experts who could help the practice. Think about how you would go about recruiting them and the implications for confidentiality.

Find out what patients think would be useful – ask for feedback, organise a focus group or set up a representative local group.

You could set up evening or Saturday morning sessions with Health and Safety experts, occupational therapists and physiotherapists for anyone who wants to learn about the prevention and management of musculoskeletal disorders.

Consider holding some sessions away from practice premises (perhaps a function room at a pub or working men's club) to encourage participation by those who would not normally visit the surgery. Think about inviting a well-known local figure to one or two of the sessions to increase the impact and get some free publicity (let the local paper or TV/radio station know about the sessions).

Arrange for computer terminals or poster displays giving access to other sources of advice provided by other agencies (e.g. libraries, Citizens' Advice Bureau, the local council).

What mechanism(s) will you use to find out the answers in a meaningful way, and not just from the most opinionated or compliant? You may need to think deeply about the reliability of any method, and how representative individual patients are of your whole practice population.[10]

Aims of your personal development plan arising from the preliminary data-gathering exercise:

To learn how to:

- identify risky behaviours (e.g. standing on a chair instead of a set of steps)
- identify harmful working practices (e.g. too much pressure to enter

data in a short time, so adopting a poor working position as a result, or stationery supplies kept on high shelves)
- investigate and establish the significant causes of musculoskeletal injuries[26]
- find out other non-medical or paramedical sources of information and resources
- do a search and audit and use a spreadsheet to record your findings
- set up forms for automating the recording of incidents and clinical encounters, management and activity reports, annual report information, etc.
- identify the risk factors for common conditions and how to prevent or minimise them[21,63,64]
- identify best practice for treatment strategies and how to implement them
- identify preventive strategies for osteoporosis and set up protocols and guidelines for delegation and consistent recording
- produce patient leaflets and a newsletter
- set up information and activity sessions for staff and the public.

How might you integrate the 14 components of clinical governance into your personal development plan focusing on the topic of musculo-skeletal disorders?

Establishing a learning culture: hold regular meetings on different aspects of identification of risky practices or good practice for team members to learn new skills and information.

Managing resources and services: identify the extra resources that might be required to make the workplace safer and healthier, the skill mix required for delivering prevention and treatment messages, and the implications for other services and resources if staff are to add prevention to their diagnostic and treatment roles.

Establishing a research and development culture: set up an automatic information-gathering service about prevention and management of musculoskeletal disorders on a website; conduct a 'before and after' study of musculoskeletal disorders in the practice.

Reliable and accurate data: enter data once, consistently and correctly, and be able to retrieve it for a variety of uses and be able to compare it with other data.

Evidence-based practice and policy: find out what preventive and treatment measures and practices have worked elsewhere, and how well proven the practices are.

Confidentiality: ensure that the data is protected against unauthorised access and not passed to others without knowing the degree of confidentiality with which it will be treated. If you need details of who has had musculoskeletal disorders in order to investigate the cause, their informed consent must be obtained first.

Health gain: the prevention and effective treatment of musculoskeletal disorders reduce time off work and disability.

Coherent team: everyone needs to know best practice for the prevention and management of musculoskeletal disorders.

Audit and evaluation: follow the management of specific conditions (e.g. osteoporosis, tendinitis), and search and audit incidents in a multiplicity of ways.

Meaningful involvement of patients and the public: hold interactive sessions with patients and the public to inform them and show ways of preventing and managing musculoskeletal disorders; provide information from leaflets, computer programs and posters.

Health promotion: target health promotion with specific reminders on screen, or select specific groups for action (e.g. for rehabilitation after a fall).

Risk management: ensure that up-to-date records are kept on incidents in the practice; surveys of equipment; surveys of best (or poor) working practices.

Accountability and performance: monitor before and after interventions. Reward and celebrate good practice and suggestions.

Core requirements: could you work out a different skill mix in your practice team to provide better prevention and management of musculoskeletal disorders?

Action plan (include the objectives above, timetabled action and expected outcomes)

Who is involved? All identified staff who need to learn about the prevention and management of musculoskeletal disorders with you.

Where? Identify the sites at which training and learning will take place.

Timetabled action: Start date: . . . . . .

By 3 months: preliminary data gathered and staff involved identified.

- Skills that are already present (in your practice, in the PCO, health authority, etc.).
- Equipment and systems that are available (yours, the practice, the PCO, outside in a training venue).
- Training that can be obtained (to match your needs).
- Training that could take place (in your practice, other practice(s), at the local college or university, at other sites such as industry, distance learning, other local or distant venue).
- How it could be done (individual or group; tutor led or cascade learning).

By 6 months: review current performance.

- Are your skills being utilised in the most effective way?
- Do the building, equipment and working practices meet the specifications for the tasks you are required to perform now and those you anticipate doing in the immediate future?

By 7 months: identify solutions and associated learning needs.

- Arrange the necessary training.
- Make a business plan for any associated equipment needs.
- Arrange cover for yourself and any other staff who are involved to provide protected time for learning.
- Clarify who does what and when.
- Negotiate the changes necessary at practice meeting(s).

By 12 months: make the changes.

- Implement the new procedures.
- Obtain feedback from other staff about its impact.
- Iron out any difficulties.
- Identify any gaps in the provision.

Expected outcomes: reduction in time off work and suffering for staff and working patients; reduction in avoidable falls and injuries; fitter staff and patients; identification of patients at risk and implementation of targeted prevention (e.g. from osteoporosis or falls, or from occupational hazards); reduction of pain and suffering; improved psychosocial status for those with chronic conditions.

How does your personal development plan tie in with your other strategic plans? (e.g. the practice's business or development plan, the local health improvement programme or the primary care investment plan?)

Make sure that your objectives mesh with theirs. They may have a priority for the prevention of osteoporosis, or the development of shared protocols for the management of musculoskeletal disorders between primary and secondary care, into which you can feed your personal development plan.

What additional resources will you require to execute your plan and from where do you hope to obtain them?

Your entitlement to reimbursement of course fees, etc., will depend on your contract and on the priority value that the practice or PCO puts on your development plan to meet their own needs.

Any additional equipment, alterations to the use of the building, working practices, etc., will have to be decided on the same basis.

How will you evaluate your learning plan?

Look at the methods you used to identify your learning needs. How does it all fit? Can you repeat a measure that you adopted to establish your learning needs to determine how much you have learned or the extent to which your performance has improved?

How will you know when you have achieved your objectives?

You will be able to carry out the tasks you have set yourself, or you will have implemented the changes specified in your list of objectives.

How will you disseminate the learning from the plan to the rest of the practice team and patients? How will you sustain your new-found knowledge or skills?

You might let everyone know by writing an article in a practice newsletter. Let the staff know what has been achieved or what is now available at team meetings.

Pass on your skills to other people in the team as required, and keep using your skills to provide information or better working practices. You could run an in-house training session to teach others in the practice team how to do one of the new procedures you have mastered (e.g. search and audit).

How will you handle new learning requirements as they crop up?

Keep a record as they arise to consider later, or add them in if they are essential at this stage.

Check whether the topic you have chosen is a priority and the way in which you plan to learn about it is appropriate.

> **Your topic:** *prevention and management of musculoskeletal disorders*

How have you identified your learning need(s)?

(*a*) PCO requirement	☒	(*e*) Appraisal need	☐
(*b*) Practice business plan	☒	(*f*) New to post	☐
(*c*) Legal mandatory require- ment (Health and Safety)	☒	(*g*) Individual decision	☐
		(*h*) Patient feedback	☐
(*d*) Job requirement	☒	(*i*) Other	☐

Have you discussed or planned your learning needs with anyone else?

Yes ☒ No ☐ If so, who? *Other staff; PCO tutor and clinical governance lead.*

What are your learning need(s) and/or objective(s) in terms of the following?

Knowledge. What new information do you hope to gain to help you to do this?

To learn how to implement strategies for the prevention and management of musculoskeletal disorders.

Skills. What should you be able to do differently as a result of undertaking this learning in your development plan?

Identify best working practices; correct poor working practices; identify risky situations; identify at-risk groups and implement prevention.

Behaviour/professional practice. How will this impact on the way in which you then do things?

Regular reviews of potential hazards; regular reviews of standards of care for at-risk groups.

Details and date of desired development activity:

Within three months: collect sufficient information. Within six months: start to implement changes to working practices and management of at-risk groups with information and interactive sessions with those patients and staff and with the wider public.

Details of any previous training and/or experience you have in this area/dates:

Piecemeal self-instruction without structure or specific objectives.

What is your current performance in this area compared with the requirements of your job?

Need significant development in this area	☒	Need some development in this area	☐
Satisfactory in this area	☐	Do well in this area	☐

What is the level of job relevance that this area has to your role and responsibilities?

Has no relevance to job	☐	Has some relevance	☐
Relevant to job	☐	Very relevant	☒
Essential to job	☐		

Describe how the proposed education/training is relevant:

Integral part of my work in the practice team.

Do you need additional support in identifying a suitable development activity?

Yes ☒   No ☐

What do you need?

To know when and where relevant sessions of training are being held. Help in accessing the basic information. Help with setting up staff, patient and public sessions.

Describe the differences or improvements for you, your practice, PCO and/or employing NHS trust as a result of undertaking this activity:

I will be able to evaluate the working practices, standards of equipment and premises, standards of prevention and management, and monitor performance and assess progress towards targets set by the practice team and PCO.

Assess the priority of your proposed educational/training activity:

Urgent ☐   High ☒   Medium ☐   Low ☐

Describe how the proposed activity will meet your learning needs rather than any other type of course or training on the topic:

A multidisciplinary approach is needed because the subject encompasses so many disciplines and areas of clinical and non-clinical work.

If you had a free choice, would you want to learn this?   Yes/No

If **No**, why not? (please circle all that apply):

Waste of time
I have already done it
It is not relevant to my work or career goals
Other

If **Yes**, what reasons are most important to you? (put them in rank order):

To improve my performance	1
To increase my knowledge	2
To get promotion	
I am just interested in it	
To be better than my colleagues	
To do a more interesting job	
To enable me to be more confident	3
Because it will help me	4

Record of your learning about the prevention of musculoskeletal disorders

You would add the date, length of time spent, etc., for each learning activity

	Activity 1 – knowledge of best practice in prevention and management of musculoskeletal disorders suffered at work	*Activity 2 – preventive activities with the practice team*	*Activity 3 – setting up public sessions*	*Activity 4 – setting up a search and audit for prevention and management of osteoporosis in at-risk groups*
In-house formal learning	An evaluation of working practices followed by a workshop run by an experienced Health and Safety expert	An occupational therapist attends to run a workshop on best working practices		A learning session on the identification of at-risk groups for osteoporosis. Protected time for other practice team members to learn consistent data entry and the reasons for it
External courses	Sessions with occupational therapist and physiotherapist		Attendance at a course on public involvement	A course on learning the relevant computer skills
Informal and personal	Observation of working practices. Recording of physical hazards (e.g. trailing leads, uneven or slippery floors, etc.). Observation of how people can adapt their working practices	Discussion with staff about their job descriptions and the improvements needed in their physical working environment	Talking to others who had done this before; involving the health visitors and local councillors	Informal sessions with team members on osteoporosis prevention and management. Help to set up an exercise programme for residents in a residential home
Qualifications and/ or experience gained?	Experiences of others at the sessions; recording of best/ poor practices	Experience in running workshops; drawing up proposals with financial implications to meet the need for improvements in the physical working environment	Experience in public participation and liaison with non-medical and paramedical sources of help	Understanding of the risk factors for osteoporosis; repeatable audit of standards for identification and preventive and management strategies

CHAPTER 14

Draw up your practice personal and professional development plan

The practice personal and professional development plan (PPDP) should cater for everyone who works in the practice. Clinical governance principles will balance the development needs of the population, the practice, the PCO and the practice team members' personal development plans (PDPs).

You might want to start by identifying your own learning needs, combining them with those of other people and then checking them against the practice business plan. Alternatively, you could start from the other direction, by developing a practice-based personal and professional development plan from your business plan and then identifying your individual learning needs within that. Whichever direction you start from, you must ensure that you integrate the needs of practice team members with those of your practice and the needs and directives of the NHS.

Your learning plan should complement the professional development both of other individuals and of the practice. If you are working on a project that involves change for other people as well as yourself, it is better to work together towards a common goal and to co-ordinate multiprofessional learning across traditional boundaries. Multiprofessional learning does not mean sitting together all learning the same information, but rather that you all learn together and individually as appropriate to your roles and responsibilities. Then all of the practice team members will understand and respect each other's contributions to the provision of co-ordinated patient-centred care.

If you work in a number of different roles or posts, gaps and duplication of activities should be avoided. After reflection about the boundaries between your roles, you may be able to focus your learning so that meeting your needs in one role benefits another.

Make your learning plan flexible. You may want to add something in later when circumstances suddenly change or an additional need becomes apparent – perhaps as a result of a complaint or hearing something new at a meeting.

Long-term locums (more than six months, say), assistants, retained doctors and salaried GPs should all be included in the practice plan. Remember to include all of those staff who work for the practice, however few their hours – you cannot manage without them or they would not be there!

Time is one of the resources that must be considered when drawing up your action plan. Adequate resources must be in place for your learning needs, and protected time must be built in.

Template for your practice personal and professional development plan

Photocopy the following pages and complete one chart per topic.

What topic have you chosen?

Who chose it?

Justify why the topic is a priority:

  (i) *A personal or professional priority?*

  (ii) *A practice priority?*

  (iii) *A district priority?*

  (iv) *A national priority?*

Who will be included in your practice personal and professional development plan?
(GPs, employed staff, attached staff, others from outside the practice, patients?)

What baseline information will you collect and how?

How will you identify your learning needs?
(How will you obtain this information and who will do it? Self-completion check-lists, discussion, appraisal, audit, patient feedback?)

What are the learning needs of the practice and how do they match individual team members' needs?

Is there any patient or public input to your practice personal and professional development plan?

Aims of your practice personal and professional development plan arising from the preliminary data-gathering exercise:

**How might you integrate the 14 components of clinical govern-
ance into your practice personal and professional development
plan, focusing on the topic of . . . . ?**

Establishing a learning culture:

Managing resources and services:

Establishing a research and development culture:

Reliable and accurate data:

Evidence-based practice and policy:

Confidentiality:

Health gain:

Coherent team:

Audit and evaluation:

Meaningful involvement of patients and the public:

Health promotion:

Risk management:

Accountability and performance:

Core requirements:

Action plan (include the objectives above, timetabled action and expected outcomes)

How does your practice personal and professional development plan tie in with your other strategic plans?
(e.g. the practice's business or development plan, the local health improvement programme and the primary care investment plan)?

What additional resources will you require to execute your plan and from where do you hope to obtain them?
(e.g. will you have to pay any course fees? Will you be able to organise any protected time for learning in working hours?)

How will you evaluate your practice personal and professional development plan?

How will you know when you have achieved your objectives?
(How will you measure success?)

How will you disseminate the learning from your plan to the rest of your team and patients? How will you sustain your new-found knowledge or skills?

How will you handle new learning requirements as they crop up?

Record of the practice team learning

Write in the topic, date and time spent for each type of learning

	Activity 1	Activity 2	Activity 3	Activity 4
In-house formal learning				
External courses				
Informal and personal				
Qualifications and/or experience gained				

Worked example of a practice personal and professional development plan: prevention and management of osteoporosis

Who chose the topic?

Many of the practice team realise that improving the care of patients with osteoporosis is of increasing importance after the preliminary learning needs assessment described in the first section of this book. The district or PCO is undertaking a strategic review of provision of services for the prevention and treatment of osteoporosis following the introduction of an open access DEXA-scanner at the local hospital. Inconsistent referral criteria and patchy provision for the identification of at-risk groups has been revealed so far.

Why is the topic a priority?

(i) *A practice and professional priority*? Good risk management is an essential part of care at a clinical level for individuals with osteoporosis. Risk management is also important from an organisational perspective in identifying those at risk, and new cases, and monitoring their continuing care. Therefore investing time and effort in improving the care of those with osteoporosis should produce tangible and significant health gains for individual patients.

(ii) *A district priority*? Several districts have set up schemes to improve the identification of at-risk groups and have local initiatives to improve the management of those with osteoporosis and more 'seamless' care across the primary/secondary care interface.

(iii) *A national priority*? The cost of the effects of osteoporosis is high. Effective prevention is cost-effective to the NHS, through avoiding fractures and disability and reducing dependency and care costs. The Department of Health has endorsed the new guidelines for the management of osteoporosis.[17,18]

Who will be included in the practice-based personal and professional development plan?

You might include the following:

- patients with osteoporosis, and their families
- GPs

- practice nurses
- health visitors
- district nurses
- physiotherapists
- occupational therapists
- community pharmacists
- practice manager
- reception staff
- National Osteoporosis Society representative
- National Carers' Association
- residential and nursing home managers.

Who will collect the baseline information and how?

A receptionist/computer operator could conduct an electronic search in your practice to identify individuals with osteoporosis and the risk factors (e.g. steroid use, oophorectomy, fragility fractures, wheelchair use, etc.), if appropriately coded. Otherwise it will be laborious to set up an at-risk register from paper records, repeat prescriptions, recall, etc. Once you know who your at-risk patients are, you can audit their care and see what you need to learn.

The local public health department at your health authority should be able to supply data about morbidity and mortality rates in your district. They may also have national data on file about the average numbers per 1000 members of the population who might be expected to have osteoporosis, categorised according to age, gender and ethnic group, or you could obtain this information from your local medical library.

The local hospital trust could give you routine and acute data about referrals and admissions of patients with osteoporosis or fragility fractures. The hospital audit department may have undertaken work on osteoporosis prior to the provision of the DEXA-scanning equipment, and might give you a breakdown of results identifying your patient or PCO populations.

Where are you now? (baseline)

- Establish how many patients with osteoporosis you have, set up criteria for identifying at-risk groups and list them by age groups.
- Compare your practice protocol for managing osteoporosis with a protocol cited in the literature as 'best practice' or a recommended district protocol or guideline.[17,18,27] If you do not have a practice protocol, write one or adopt someone else's.

- Find out how many patients attend follow-up appointments in line with your practice protocol – for the various groups with osteoporosis, different age groups or ethnic groups. Work out whether you need to make follow-up appointments more available or convenient.
- Determine how good treatment is in your patients with established DEXA-scan confirmed osteoporosis. How many of them have improved bone density after treatment?
- Focus on prevention of avoidable risks (e.g. looking at the number who eat a diet low in calcium, have little exposure to sunlight, smoke or take little exercise).
- Assess the quantity and quality of literature available for patients and their families in your practice.
- Review the extent of education or training that the clinical staff have received about osteoporosis.
- Undertake an analysis of the strengths, weaknesses, opportunities and threats (SWOT) of your practice team in managing and preventing osteoporosis and other musculoskeletal disorders.

What information will you obtain about individual learning wishes and needs?

You might review the practice protocol and baseline information with as many staff as possible at a discussion group and find out whether they feel competent as individuals to carry out their roles and responsibilities, or if they want to realign their duties. They might comment on how well others are fulfilling their responsibilities and suggest improvements to the systems or procedures that have educational and resource consequences (e.g. training sessions, new equipment, effects on other parts of the practice organisation).

You could conduct a significant event audit (e.g. in a patient on long-term steroids who has a fragility fracture, or someone who has had an oophorectomy but has not been assessed for osteoporosis risk and treated appropriately).

What are the learning needs for the practice and how do they match the needs of the individual?

Responding to the queries from the district or PCO about the practice's management of osteoporosis might reveal inadequacies in your baseline knowledge of what services you are providing, how they are utilised or what you are achieving. This might create the opportunity to review how individuals contribute to the overall care provided (include the employed and attached staff as well as individuals such as the local community pharmacist or residential care home manager). Once you are sure of everyone's roles and responsibilities and your vision for the care you intend to provide, you can reassess individuals' learning needs in a co-ordinated plan to match the service that you will provide.

Compare your own figures for the numbers of people with osteoporosis with those you would expect in a practice population of the same size and demographic make-up. Decide whether you need to be more pro-active in identifying at-risk groups or new cases of osteoporosis, and address lack of knowledge or skills, uncaring attitudes or inadequate systems.

Compare prescribing patterns (current PACT data) between the GPs in your practice, and with other practices. Look for differences and inconsistencies that may indicate learning needs.

A patient complaint may reveal learning needs for individuals or the practice organisation (e.g. from the relatives of a 60-year-old woman about the delay in detecting her osteoporotic vertebral collapse).

Compare your practice protocol for the management of osteoporosis with other recommended guidelines in order to reveal learning needs.

The practice nurse or health visitor might have nominated osteoporosis as a topic that they wished to learn more about, at their annual job appraisal.[5,7] If no one else in the practice has expert knowledge or skills in the management of osteoporosis, then it would be well worth the practice facilitating the nurse to attend an in-depth course.

The practice manager may be new to the area and intend to visit other practices to learn the ropes, and he or she might take a particular interest in observing how other practices manage their services for the prevention and treatment of osteoporosis. This focus might justify additional time spent on practice visiting.

Is there any patient or public input to your plan?

Ask the relatives or patients who made a complaint or comment to help you to devise better systems in the practice or write an account of their experiences that can be used for an in-house training session.

You might ask the local representative of the National Osteoporosis Society or a patient with osteoporosis to attend an informal training session, in particular dealing with educating and informing patients better, motivating patients about prevention of risks, and informing them about side-effects of treatment.

An open evening on osteoporosis that is held for patients with osteoporosis and those at-risk, together with their relatives, will provide an opportunity for patients to mix with GPs, nurses, therapists, orthotists and non-clinical staff. Informal conversations during the evening should reveal learning needs and ideas for improvements.

Aims of the practice personal and professional development plan arising from the preliminary data-gathering exercise

After gathering baseline data and undertaking a preliminary learning needs assessment, you might design a practice personal and professional development plan that has a grand overarching aim to develop a learning programme for all members of the practice team, attached staff and individuals (e.g. the community pharmacists or managers of residential and nursing homes) to enable them to provide effective prevention and management of osteoporosis within the available resources.

Alternatively, you might concentrate on developing particular key individuals (e.g. a GP or practice nurse or specific receptionist) with lead responsibility for the clinical management or practice organisation for the prevention and treatment of osteoporosis. They could then cascade their learning in-house to others in the practice team.

As another option, you could focus down on aspects of the effective management of osteoporosis. For instance, to develop a learning programme for all members of the wider primary healthcare team to increase their knowledge and skills in educating and informing patients and their families about the prevention of osteoporosis. This might include learning how to motivate patients to comply with recommended management practices, avoid risks and complications, and comply with treatment.

How might you integrate the 14 components of clinical governance into your practice personal and professional development plan focusing on the prevention and management of osteoporosis?

Establishing a learning culture: a multidisciplinary team might update their learning about the risk factors for osteoporosis. The practice manager could learn about setting up systems for detecting new cases of osteoporosis, facilitating follow-up care and encouraging compliance. The nurses and GPs could learn about management and better ways to motivate patients to comply with treatment.

Managing resources and services: promote close working relationships and teamwork between the practice-employed staff, independent contractors such as the community pharmacist, and trust-employed staff such as physiotherapists.

Establishing a research and development culture: encourage practice team members to critically appraise published papers describing new findings in osteoporosis, in order to check whether the results described are applicable to their population.

Reliable and accurate data: keep good records to enable active follow-up of any patients with osteoporosis who are unable to get to the surgery, such as the housebound, or others who fail to attend at regular intervals.

Evidence-based practice and policy: the practice protocol for patients with different risk factors for osteoporosis should be based on the best evidence for the population and local circumstances.

Confidentiality: there should be water-tight systems in place to prevent any information about a patient with osteoporosis or risk factors for the latter being released without their consent. Any issues of confidentiality should be clarified before information about individuals is passed to others.

Health gain: good compliance with treatment by patients reduces the risk of complications from osteoporosis.

Coherent team: all members of the practice team should understand each other's roles and responsibilities in providing care.

Audit and evaluation: a significant event audit (e.g. of a patient with risk factors suffering a fragility fracture) should indicate areas where further training is required, or where practice services and teamwork need to be improved.

Meaningful involvement of patients and the public: you might hold a public session demonstrating strategies for preventing osteoporosis. This could be held in the surgery and attended by representatives from the voluntary sector, as well as patients, clinicians and staff from health and leisure clubs. A focus group of patients with osteoporosis might reveal flaws in staff knowledge and attitudes, or malfunctioning practice systems.

Health promotion: target patients at risk of osteoporosis with advice about their lifestyle, especially diet, exercise and the role of treatment.

Risk management: identification and control of risks are the main aims for the prevention and management of osteoporosis, to reduce the likelihood and extent of disability, dependence or premature death.

Accountability and performance: demonstrate that the advice and treatment that staff are providing to patients with risk factors for, or established, osteoporosis are in line with best practice.

Core requirements: practice staff should be competent and trained for the roles and responsibilities that are delegated to them by the GPs and practice manager.

Action plan (include timetabled action and expected outcomes)

Who is involved? Staff as set out previously – specify names and posts.

Where? Identify the sites at which learning will take place (e.g. hospital, practice, etc.).

Timetabled action. Start date: . . . . .

By 3 months: preliminary data-gathering and collate details of potential sources of help and training.

- Is there a practice protocol or guide on effective prevention and management of osteoporosis?
- Numbers of staff; map expertise; list other providers.
- Referral patterns for routine advice and monitoring of osteoporosis, admissions with fractures or to residential or nursing care, for advice/ help for complications.
- Information about the characteristics of those recorded on the practice computer as having osteoporosis (e.g. age group, ethnic origin).
- Any relevant local and national priorities, and any additional asso- ciated resources for which you might apply.
- Staff discussion to report problems that limit patients with osteo- porosis of different age groups, etc. accessing services, the problems, and their views and suggestions.

By 4 months: review current performance.

- Practice manager reviews operation of services and closeness of working relationships with those in other organisations and sectors who have an interest in or responsibility for the prevention and management of osteoporosis.
- Clinical leads (e.g. GP, nurse) review the extent of knowledge, skills and attitudes of the practice team with regard to the prevention and management of osteoporosis.
- Audit actual performance vs. pre-agreed criteria (e.g. with regard to referrals, education given to those with risk factors for or established osteoporosis, and investigations, monitoring and compliance or concordance).
- Compare performance with any or several of the 14 components of clinical governance (e.g. health promotion would be very relevant).

By 6 months: identify solutions and associated training needs.

- Set up new systems for access to services appropriate to the prevention and management of osteoporosis.
- Give the practice team in-house training on important aspects of the prevention and management of osteoporosis.
- Revise the practice protocol. Address identified gaps in care, having undertaken a search for other evidence-based protocols. Agree on roles and responsibilities as a team for delivering care and services according to the protocol; arrange for certain staff to attend external courses. The practice or district nurse, GP, pharmacist, or rheumatologist could provide some in-house training to GPs and nurses, the community pharmacist or others from outside organisations with whom the practice is liaising about the issue.

By 12 months: make changes.

- Clinicians adhere to practice protocol as shown by repeat audits and patient feedback.
- change service times and locations to make them more appropriate for those with osteoporosis of various age groups, disabilities and ethnic groups, having organised training to anticipate new requirements (e.g. train residential and nursing-home managers to give the same advice as other members of the primary care team).

Expected outcomes: more effective prevention and management of osteoporosis; better patient compliance with treatment and good lifestyle habits; fewer fragility fractures; more patients with risk factors being able to live independently.

How does your practice personal and professional development plan tie in with your other strategic plans?

The practice's business plan and the PCO's primary care investment plan might both prioritise the achievement of more effective prevention and management of osteoporosis. The practice personal and professional development plan that focuses on the prevention and management of osteoporosis would complement those strategic plans.

What additional resources will you require to execute your plan and from where do you hope to obtain them?

The practice might pay for the course fees of any member of staff who undertakes training that fulfils a priority need of the practice.

You may be able to justify an application for additional resources to your PCO, health authority or local NHS trust with your preliminary learning and health needs assessments, tapping into the district or national strategic priorities. You could point out that this expenditure would be balanced by savings from the prevention of fractures in patients with osteoporosis.

If a member of staff is undertaking the training on behalf of the practice, you should try to arrange that the training is undertaken within paid time. Any learning that is cascaded to other members of the practice team as part of the practice personal and professional development plan should also be undertaken in paid time and during working hours whenever possible.

How will you evaluate your practice personal and professional development plan?

You should be able to select methods of evaluation from the range of methods suggested for assessing learning needs in the reflective exercises. The most appropriate methods will depend on the specific aims that you set for your practice personal and professional development plan. For example, if your main aim is to prevent osteoporosis in people with medical risk factors, you might evaluate this by monitoring all patients on long-term steroids and with sex-hormone deficiencies. However, if your aim was to improve the levels and appropriateness of education and information for people with environmental risk factors for osteoporosis, you might evaluate your achievements by asking the patients themselves – by a simple test of knowledge, focus-group discussion of experiences, monitoring changes in patient behaviour, etc.

The practice manager and clinical lead for the prevention and management of osteoporosis (e.g. GP or practice nurse) might plan the evaluation together and delegate the collection of data to a receptionist.

How will you know when you have achieved your objectives?

Usually you will determine this by comparing the outcomes of your programme with baseline data. However, it might also be determined by looking at patients' compliance with recommended practice, or the lifestyle changes that they have achieved.

How will you disseminate the learning from the plan to the rest of the practice team and patients? How will you sustain your new-found knowledge and skills?

You might write about it in a practice newsletter. Let all the staff know at practice meetings what progress has been made. You might want to describe your success at a PCO meeting or apply for an award for best practice from one of the national GP newspapers. Pass on your skills and knowledge to others as required, and review your protocol at set intervals in order to incorporate new information.

How will you handle new learning requirements as they crop up?

The practice manager might run audits at intervals and feed the results back to a practice meeting mid-way through the time period of the practice personal and professional development plan, when there is time to revise the activities.

Record of practice team learning about the prevention and management of oseoporosis

You would add the date, length of time spent etc., for each learning activity

	Activity 1 – revise practice protocol	Activity 2 – update patient education	Activity 3 – identification of osteoporosis	Activity 4 – preventing complications of osteoporosis
In-house formal learning	Practice team discussion of roles and responsibilities of various members to fulfil protocol, including district nurses and the community pharmacist	A pharmaceutical representative shows a non-promotional video on educating patients with risk factors for osteoporosis, which is watched by GPs, nurses and the community pharmacist	GP and nurse with new ideas on targeting and detecting (see below) share their ideas with the rest of the practice team during practice discussion of osteoporosis protocol (see Activity 1)	Hospital specialist input to follow-up practice team discussion when changes to practice protocol are reviewed, with any changes to medication for patients with established osteoporosis or those at risk
External courses	GP/nurse lead on osteoporosis attends two-day continuing education course on osteoporosis at regional centre			Practice nurse attends a half-day course on health promotion and motivating patients, and she then extrapolates this learning to osteoporosis
Informal and personal	Practice nurse searches for examples of best practice on Medline at home. Practice manager rings up other practices to ask other practice managers if they have protocols, and discusses differences	After watching the video, the practice manager brings in all of the available literature and audio-visual aids on osteoporosis. The team sorts these according to criteria already agreed from a previous initiative on asthma	A GP attending a two-day external course and practice nurse attending local practice nurse group meeting pick up tips for targeted screening and being more alert to the possibility of osteoporosis	Practice team members all learn from talking to patients with osteoporosis in the course of their daily work how to make more impact with recommendations for a healthier lifestyle
Qualifications and/or experience gained	GP/nurse lead receives accreditation for two-day course that can be put towards a university certificate in health practice			Practice nurse's attendance at a half-day course is recorded in her own reflective portfolio for discussion with her clinical supervisor

References

1 Clarke R and Croft P (1998) *Critical Reading for the Reflective Practitioner.* Reed Educational and Professional Publishing, Butterworth-Heinemann, Oxford.

2 Chalmers I and Altman DG (1995) *Systematic Reviews.* BMJ Publishing Group, London.

3 Members of the *Ad Hoc* Committee on Clinical Guidelines (1996) Guidelines for the initial evaluation of the adult patient with acute musculoskeletal symptoms. *Arthritis Rheumatism.* **39**: 1–8.

4 Chambers R, Hawksley B, Smith G and Chambers C (2001) *Back Pain Matters in Primary Care.* Radcliffe Medical Press, Oxford.

5 Chambers R and Wakley G (2000) *Making Clinical Governance Work for You.* Radcliffe Medical Press, Oxford.

6 Lilley R (1999) *Making Sense of Clinical Governance.* Radcliffe Medical Press, Oxford.

7 Wakley G, Chambers R and Field S (2000) *Continuing Professional Development.* Radcliffe Medical Press, Oxford.

8 Royal College of General Practitioners (2000) *Access to General Practice Based Primary Care.* Royal College of General Practitioners, London.

9 Dunning M, Abi-Aad G, Gilbert D *et al.* (1999) *Experience, Evidence and Everyday Practice.* King's Fund, London.

10 Chambers R (2000) *Involving Patients and Public.* Radcliffe Medical Press, Oxford.

11 Department of Health (1997) Report of the review of patient-identifiable information. In: *The Caldicott Committee Report.* Department of Health, London.

12 Schoenbaum S and Gottlieb L (1990) Algorithm-based improvement of clinical quality. *BMJ.* **301**: 1374–6.

13 Hurwitz B (1998) *Clinical Guidelines and the Law.* Radcliffe Medical Press, Oxford.

14 Muir Gray JA (1997) *Evidence-Based Healthcare.* Churchill Livingstone, Edinburgh.

15 Barton S (ed.) (2001) *Clinical Evidence. Issue 5.* BMJ Publishing Group, London.

16 Donald P (2000) Promoting the local ownership of guidelines. *Guidelines Pract.* **3**: 17.

17 Royal College of Physicians (1999) *Osteoporosis. Clinical guidelines for prevention and treatment.* Royal College of Physicians, London.

18 Royal College of Physicians, Bone and Tooth Society of Great Britain (2000) *Osteoporosis. Clinical guidelines for prevention and treatment. Update of pharmacological interventions and an algorithm for management.* Royal College of Physicians, London.

19 Messier SP, Loeser RF, Mitchell MN *et al.* (2000) Exercise and weight loss in obese older adults with knee osteoarthritis: a preliminary study. *J Am Geriatr Soc.* **48**: 1062–72.

20 Helliwell PS and O'Hara M (1995) Shared care between hospital and general practice: an audit of disease-modifying drug monitoring in rheumatoid arthritis. *Br J Rheumatol.* **34**: 673–6.

21 Chambers R, Moore S, Parker G and Slovak A (2001) *Occupational Health Matters in General Practice.* Radcliffe Medical Press, Oxford.

22 Mohanna K and Chambers R (2000) *Risk Matters: communicating risk and clinical risk management.* Radcliffe Medical Press, Oxford.

23 Multidisciplinary Development Group (2000) *Learning Guide for General Practitioners and General Practitioner Registrars.* Arthritis and Rheumatism Campaign, Chesterfield.

24 Michael McGhee M (2000) *A Guide to Laboratory Investigations* (3e). Radcliffe Medical Press, Oxford.

25 Dieppe P and Payne T (1994) Referral guidelines for general practitioners – which patients with limb joint arthritis should be sent to a rheumatologist? *ARC Rep Rheumatic Dis: Series 3.* **1**: 1–7.

26 Snaith ML (ed.) (1999) *ABC of Rheumatology.* BMJ Books, London.

27 Foord-Kelcey G (ed.) (2000) *Guidelines Volume 12.* Medenium Group Publishing Ltd, Berkhamstead.

28 Altman R, Brandt K, Hochberg M *et al.* (1996) Design and conduct of clinical trials in patients with osteoarthritis: recommendations from a task force of the Osteoarthritis Research Society. *Osteoarthritis Cartilage.* **4**: 217–43.

29 Madhok R, Kerr H and Capell HA (2000) Recent advances: rheumatology. *BMJ.* **321**: 882–5.

30 Watson MC, Brookes ST, Kirwan JR and Faulkner A (2000) Non-aspirin, non-steroidal anti-inflammatory drugs for osteoarthritis of the knee (Cochrane Review) In: *The Cochrane Library. Issue 3.* Update Software, Oxford.

31 Towheed T, Shea B, Wells G and Hochberg M (2000) Analgesia and non-aspirin, non-steroidal anti-inflammatory drugs for osteoarthritis of the hip (Cochrane Review) In: *The Cochrane Library. Issue 3.* Update Software, Oxford.

32 Hardom DC and Holmes AC (1997) The New Zealand priority criteria project. *BMJ.* **314**: 131–4.

33 March LM, Cross MJ, Lapsley H *et al.* (1999) Outcomes after hip or knee replacement surgery for osteoarthritis. A prospective cohort study comparing patients' quality of life before and after surgery with age-related norms. *Med J Austr.* **171**: 235–8.

34 van Essen GJ, Chipchase LS, O'Connor D and Krishnan J (1998) Primary

total knee replacement: short term outcomes in an Australian population. *J Qual Clin Pract.* **18**: 135–42.

35 Irvine D and Irvine S (1991) *Making Sense of Audit.* Radcliffe Medical Press, Oxford.

36 Perkins P and Jones AC (1999) Gout. *Ann Rheumatic Dis.* **58**: 611–16.

37 Klippel J, Dieppe P and Ferri F (1999) *Primary Care Rheumatology.* Mosby, London.

38 Davis JC (1999) A practical approach to gout: current management of an old disease. *Postgrad Med.* **106**: 115–23.

39 NSAID Focus (1998) June *Bandolier* available on http://www.jr2.ox.ac.uk/bandolier/band52/b52–2.html

40 Symmonds DP, Barrett EM, Bankhead CR, Scott DG and Silman AJ (1994) The incidence of rheumatoid arthritis in the United Kingdom: results from the Norfolk Arthritis Register. *Br J Rheumatol.* **33**: 735–9.

41 Yelin E, Henke C and Epstein W (1987) The work dynamic of the person with rheumatoid arthritis. *Arthritis Rheumatism.* **30**: 507–12.

42 Mutru O, Laakso M, Isom ki H and Koota K (1985) Ten-year mortality and causes of death in patients with rheumatoid arthritis. *BMJ.* **290**: 1811–13.

43 Felson DT, Anderson JJ, Boers M *et al.* (1995) American College of Rheumatology preliminary definition of improvement in rheumatoid arthritis. *Arthritis Rheumatism.* **38**: 727–35.

44 By permission from Wolstanton Medical Practice, Palmerston Street, Newcastle-under-Lyme, Staffordshire ST5 8BN.

45 American College of Rheumatology Guidelines Committee (1996) Guidelines for rheumatoid arthritis management. *Arthritis Rheumatism.* **39**: 713–22.

46 Collier J (ed.) (2000) Managing falls in older people. *Drug Ther Bull.* **38**: 68–72.

47 National Osteoporosis Society, PO Box 10, Radstock, Bath BA3 3YB. Patient helpline 01761 472721.

48 Mehta DK *et al.* (March, 2001) *British National Formulary.* BMA and The Royal Pharmaceutical Society of Great Britain, London.

49 Compston J (2000) Updated guidelines on osteoporosis, including management algorithm. *Guidelines Pract.* **3**: 23–8.

50 Goudz BA (2000) Whiplash injury. *Am J Nursing.* **100**: 41.

51 Silver T (1998) *Joint and Soft Tissue Injection.* Radcliffe Medical Press, Oxford.

52 The Disability Partnership (1999) *One in Four of Us (experience disability).* The Disability Partnership, London.

53 Martin J, Meltzer H and Elliot D (1988–89) *OPCS Survey of Disability in Great Britain. Six reports.* HMSO, London.

54 Munday S (1997) *Medical Education in Relation to Disability and Rehabilitation.* The Disability Partnership, London.

55 Royal Pharmaceutical Society of Great Britain (1997) *From Compliance to Concordance: towards shared goals in medicine taking.* Royal Pharmaceutical Society of Great Britain, London.

56 Heath I (1995) *The Mystery of General Practice.* Nuffield Provincial Hospitals Trust, London.

57 Dieppe P (1991) *An Introduction to the Musculoskeletal System: a handbook for medical students.* Arthritis Research Campaign, Chesterfield.

58 Jenkinson C and McGee H (1998) *Health Status Measurement: a brief but critical introduction.* Radcliffe Medical Press, Oxford.

59 Department of Social Security (2000) *Guidance for Doctors. 1B204 guide.* Department of Social Security, London.

60 Health and Safety Executive (1998) *Good Health is Good Business: an employer's guide.* HSE Books, Sudbury.

61 Kloss D (1998) *Occupational Health Law* (3e). Blackwell Science, Oxford.

62 *The Disability Discrimination Act 1995.* The Stationery Office, London.

63 Cooper C, Snow S, McAlindon TE *et al.* (2000) Risk factors for the incidence and progression of radiographic knee osteoarthritis. *Arthritis Rheumatism.* **43**: 995–1000.

64 Coggon D, Croft P, Kellingray S *et al.* (2000) Occupational physical activities and osteoarthritis of the knee. *Arthritis Rheumatism.* **43**: 1443–9.

Sources of help

Useful addresses

Arthritis and Rheumatism Council, St Mary's Court, St Mary's Gate, Chesterfield, Derbyshire S41 7TD. Tel: 01246 558033.

British League Against Rheumatism, 41 Eagle Street, London WC1R 4AR. Tel: 020 7242 3313.

Lupus UK, 51 North Street, Romford, Essex RM1 1BA. Tel: 01708 731251.

National Osteoporosis Society, PO Box 10, Radstock, Bath BA3 3YB. Tel: 01761 471771.

Primary Care Rheumatology Society, PO Box 42, Northallerton, North Yorkshire DL7 8YG.

Useful websites

Note that websites often change or disappear.

On guidelines

Agency for Health Care Policy and Research (AHCPR)	http://www.guideline.gov
Bandolier	http://ebandolier.com
Canadian Medical Association	http://www.cma.ca/cpgs/
Cochrane Collaboration	http://www.cochrane.org
*e*Guidelines	http://www.eguidelines.co.uk
General Medical Council	http://www.gmc-uk.org
Guideline Appraisal Project	http://www.cche.net/principles/content_all.asp
Guideline Project	http://www.ihs.ox.ac.uk/guidelines/
HoN (Health on the Net)	http://www.hon.ch

Medline	http://www.omni.ac.uk/medline
New Zealand Guidelines Group	http://www.nzgg.org.nz
NLM Health Services/Technology Assessment	http://www.nlm.nih.gov
North of England Evidence Based Guidelines	http://www.ncl.ac.uk/~ncenthsr/ publicn/guide/guide.htm
OMNI (Organising Medical Networked Information)	http://www.omni.ac.uk
Primary Care Online	http://www.primarycareonline.co.uk
PRODIGY	http://www.prodigy.nhs.uk
Scottish Intercollegiate Guidelines Network (SIGN)	http://www.sign.ac.uk
St George's Health Care Evaluation Unit	http://www.sghms.ac.uk/depts/phs/ hceu/nhsguide.htm
UK Health Centre	http://www.healthcentre.org.uk/hc/ library/guidelines.htm
WISDOM Centre	http://www.wisdomnet.co.uk

On musculoskeletal disorders

American College of Rheumatology	http://www.rheumatology.org
Arthritis Research Campaign	http://www.arc.org.uk
Arthritis Resource Centre	http://www.healingwell.com/ arthritis
Birmingham University	http://rheumb.bham.ac.uk
British Medical Journal	http://www.bmj.com
British Society for Rheumatology and British League against Rheumatism	http://www.rheumatology.org.uk
Current Problems in Pharmacovigilance	http://www.open.gov.uk
Doctor's Desk	http://drsdesk.sghms.ac.uk
International League of Associations for Rheumatology	http://www.ilar.org
Lancet	http://www.thelancet.com
National Electronic Library for Health	http://nelh.nhs.uk
National Osteoporosis Society	http://www.noc.org.uk
Rheumatology Web	http://www.rheumatologyweb.com
Royal College of Physicians Guidelines	http://www.open.gov/osteop.htm
Sheffield University	http://www.shef.ac.uk/uni/ projects/mc

Index